Pregnancy and Childbirth

Expecting a Baby Pregnancy Guide

Pregnancy What to Expect Pregnancy Health

Pregnancy Eating and Recipes

By Cheri Merz and John McArthur

Copyright

ISBN-13:978-1495937712

ISBN-10:1495937712

Natural Health Magazine

www.naturalhealthmagazine.net

The information in this book is provided for educational and information purposes only. It is not intended to be used as medical advice or as a substitute for treatment by a doctor or healthcare provider.

The information and opinions contained in this publication are believed to be accurate based on the information available to the author. However, the contents have not been evaluated by the U.S. Food and Drug Administration and are not intended to diagnose, treat, cure or prevent disease.

Warning

Table of Contents

Copyright..2

Introduction 10

Before you attempt to conceive... 11

Conception tips 18

    A little biology lesson................................... 18

You think you're pregnant: what's next?..................... 23

    Signs and symptoms 23

    Menstrual period late.................................. 23

    Morning sickness 26

    Fatigue... 28

    Breast changes.. 30

    Frequent urination.................................... 32

    Abdominal cramping and pressure.................... 32

    Headaches... 33

    Mood swings 34

    Food cravings 35

Finding your medical professionals **37**

What to expect at your first appointment 39

Future Appointments 41

Healthy pregnancy lifestyle **42**

Nutrition 44

Macronutrients.. 46

Five food groups.. 48

Other nutritional considerations............................ 49

3 Very important tips 50

Supplements 50

Foods to avoid.. 51

Seafood 52

Unpasteurized dairy 52

Undercooked and improperly handled foods.......... 52

Caffeine.. 53

Alcohol 54

Exercise and Other Activity 54

Your exercise program 54

Working while pregnant 56

Everyday activities 57

Sex during pregnancy 59

Healthy meals during pregnancy **61**

3 Easy breakfast recipes 61

Fresh Herb Omelet 61

Guilt-Free Breakfast Pizza 63

Delicious Oats topped with Bananas and Walnuts 64

Healthy dinner recipes 65

Curry Infused Beef Pilaf 65

Chicken and Sun-dried Tomato Pasta 67

Spicy grilled Fish and Fresh Vegetables 69

3 Quick and healthy lunch recipes 71

Delicious Chicken Tortilla 71

Turkey and Coleslaw Sandwich 73

Vegetarian Open Sandwich..74

Sweet and healthy 75

Refreshing Vanilla Yoghurt and Mango Pops.........................75

Pecan, Almond and Dried Fruit Bars 76

Mixed Berry and Banana Smoothie...................................78

Common health issues during pregnancy...........................**79**

Anemia 79

Autoimmune disorders...82

Depression 82

Diabetes 83

Thyroiditis..84

Other complaints 85

Sleeping position and stillbirth **86**

The stages of pregnancy..**88**

First trimester—weeks 1 to 12 89

Second trimester—weeks 13 to 29 91

Third trimester—weeks 30 to 41......................................92

Fetal movement 95

Labor and delivery 98

Before your due date—birthing classes 98

Before your due date—birth plan 100

What do you want to happen during a normal labor and

delivery? 101

Pre-labor symptoms 103

First-stage labor 107

Stage-two labor 111

Third-Stage Labor 115

Postpartum 116

Baby blues, postpartum depression and postpartum

psychosis 117

Postpartum perineal care 119

Postpartum care after C-section 121

Sex after pregnancy 122

Breastfeeding 124

Inverted nipples 125

Postpartum depression or psychosis.................................... 125

Contagious or infectious disease/requirement for unsafe

medication 126

Insufficient milk supply or quality.. 126

Summary.. 127

Bibliography 128

More Books by John McArthur... 129

Introduction

Pregnancy and childbirth are, to most new parents, the most exciting and joyful periods of their lives next to watching that precious bundle grow. Though to many it is a delightful surprise to find they are pregnant, many others plan and try for some time before managing to conceive.

Often, books like this start at the point where conception has taken place and offers the new mom-to-be a wealth of information about what to expect during a normal pregnancy. Don't worry, we will do that too; but we hope you have acquired this book before conception, because there are many important preparations to make for a healthy pregnancy and the best chance for your baby to be as perfect in every way as you could wish. So, this book will start with how to do exactly that—prepare for a healthy pregnancy.

Before you attempt to conceive...

Just take a quick look at your last New Year's Resolutions. Do they read something like this?

- Stop smoking
- Start an exercise program
- Eat healthier
- Lose weight

If so, you have your plan to prepare for pregnancy pre-written. All we need to do is help you find a way to keep those resolutions.

But seriously, it is important for your baby's health as well as for your own during pregnancy and later while caring for your child that you yourself be in the best health you can before becoming pregnant. Think about it for a moment, especially if this is your first baby. Do you really want to have all the same old health concerns you have always had while also being hyper-alert for anything and everything that could go wrong during your pregnancy? Most experienced moms will tell you that you absolutely do NOT want that. So let's talk about these issues.

First, any habit that your doctor would nag you about whether you were pregnant or not needs to go, not only for the baby's sake, but for yours. Do you smoke? Stop! There are numerous books, programs, supplements, even medical interventions to help do this. If you are not motivated for yourself, at least be motivated for your baby. Imagine being locked inside a smoky room with no way to escape, your lungs not developed enough to filter and expel the smoke. Your tiny tummy aches from coughing, and your lungs burn, but you can't get out. That's what it is like for your baby when you smoke while pregnant. Smoking while pregnant represents a number of risks for your baby, both before and after birth, including low birth weight, general poor health, physical and intellectual underdevelopment and even death from SIDS (Sudden Infant Death Syndrome) during the first few weeks of life. Smoking is also reported to make morning sickness worse.

Most smokers report difficulty breaking the habit...do not add to this difficulty the stress of doing it while you are also tired, cranky from hormonal changes and suffering from morning sickness! If you are already pregnant, your doctor may urge you to quit immediately, or if s/he knows you are suffering from other external stress, may tell you to stop gradually to avoid placing more stress on you. Whatever the case, the sooner you can stop smoking, the better it will be for your baby. By the way, second-hand smoke is just as bad, so new dad should also stop smoking, and new mom should avoid other smoky environments. It may even help to stop smoking if you avoid the smoke-break room or any area that triggers your desire to smoke.

The same goes for alcohol consumption. Because it is typically at least a couple of weeks before you know you are pregnant after conception (and frequently even more), you should stop consuming alcohol as soon as you start trying to conceive. No one knows how much alcohol is harmful to baby, but it IS known that babies who are exposed to alcohol in the womb are at risk from everything from low birth weight to full-blown fetal alcohol spectrum disease, which can cause heart problems, facial deformities and mental retardation in addition to introducing the baby to a painful world where she must withdraw from a poisonous substance just like an adult alcoholic.

Do we even need to talk about illicit drugs? We are going to presume that if you are concerned enough to read this book, you are not the type of person who would deliberately expose your baby to those. However, your perfectly legitimate medications could also pose a risk to baby, so before you try to conceive, you should discuss your regular medications and any herbal supplements you take regularly with your doctor. If you find that some could be harmful to your unborn child, you will want to discuss finding alternatives or withdrawing from these medications, if possible, before conception.

If you were already pregnant before you stopped using any harmful substances, but stopped as soon as you found out, rest assured that many people have gone that route without significant harm to their babies. Try not to worry, and make sure you stick to healthier habits from now on. If it took a while before you were able to stop or before you realized you were pregnant, talk to your doctor about what the substances were, when you stopped, and what steps to take if she thinks your baby may be at risk. Finding a hospital with a good NICU (Newborn Intensive Care Unit) could go a long way toward easing your mind. Worrying will not help and will only add your stress hormones to what baby has to deal with in utero, so do your best not to worry.

Now that we have discussed your bad habits, let's talk about some good ones. Good health for anyone includes a reasonably healthy diet and a reasonably active lifestyle or exercise regimen. If you feel yours could stand some improvement, it is far easier to start that now, before trying to conceive, although you probably do not have to wait to start trying the latter to improve the former. There may be more books on the subjects of eating healthier, exercising and losing weight than any other combination of subjects, so feel free to consult some of them. We would recommend, however, that you stay away from the fad 'diet' plans. Consider how many of those books there are, and how often the next 'new' thing comes along. For that matter, take a look at the fine print in the TV or internet ads for weight loss supplements—virtually all of them say that the supplement works when combined with a healthy diet and exercise. Guess what? That works, and works surprisingly quickly, without the supplement!

Here are a few tips to start your journey to better health as you prepare a healthier home for your baby for the nine months or so he is in residence. First, choose healthy foods. These include lean meats or other protein sources; lots of vegetables and some fruits; whole-grain carbohydrates like bread, cereal and flour; some healthy fats like olive oil, nuts or seeds and fatty fruits like avocado; dairy or other sources of calcium, and plenty of fresh, pure water.

Second, pay attention to portions; they are important. Learn the truth about what a serving is. For example, that bowl of whole grain cereal should have no more than ¾-1 cup of cereal in it; but the bowl might hold up to 3-4 cups. Rather than simply filling your bowl, measuring for a while helps to give you a visual of the correct serving size; or there are plenty of analogies, like 3-4 oz. of meat being about the size of a deck of playing cards. Vary your foods to provide you with plenty of what you like in reasonable portions, and you are well on your way to healthier eating.

You can even have sweets, on occasion and in modest servings. As a former yo-yo dieter, I would personally recommend you give up all sweets for several weeks, and then, only if you have great self-control, carefully re-introduce them in bite-sized servings to avoid getting back into the habit of daily over-consumption. You may be surprised at what will satisfy your sweet-tooth.

As for exercise, anyone who has been sedentary should consult a doctor to be certain they are healthy enough to start an exercise program; and if you aren't, you certainly aren't ready to conceive a child. But most people can start a moderate plan of walking daily for up to 30 minutes, combined with some body-weight strength exercises such as squats, lunges, etc. While trying to conceive, you might want to keep it very moderate or even light, especially if you are overweight as well as just generally out-of-shape. Your doctor will be your best guide to this undertaking, so follow his directions.

A word about stretching. Many books will tell you to stretch before exercise. This is NOT correct, at least not entirely. No one, especially a pregnant woman whose muscles and ligaments are subject to a hormone that encourages loosening for the birth event, should stretch before warming up. A good warm-up will prepare your muscles and ligaments to stretch without injury, so be sure you do one, either something your doctor recommends or a modified version of whatever exercise you are about to undertake; for example, a beginner might walk slowly for five minutes, stretch, then walk more briskly for up to 20 minutes, then slowly again to cool down. Stretching after your cool-down also will help you avoid sore muscles after exercise, so be sure to do that too.

Once you are pregnant, even if you already have excellent food and exercise habits, you may notice that some adjustments are required to both diet and exercise. We will address those in a later section. If you are already pregnant when you read this book, but need to follow a stricter diet or begin an exercise plan for good health, once again your doctor will be your best guide.

Conception tips

A little biology lesson

Everything you need to know about getting pregnant, you learned in seventh grade health class, right? Maybe, but not necessarily. You probably learned the basics, egg and sperm, menstrual cycle, ovulation, etc. It's what you didn't learn that we are going to cover in this section. It is the author's personal theory that there is a reason why teenagers get caught pregnant woefully often, while more mature women in their twenties and thirties, much less older, might have to try for months to conceive—birth control. This, by the way is merely an opinion, nothing that has been proven by scientific research as far as we know.

More than likely, you have been using some form of birth control for several years, and you may have skipped the information that some types of birth control can have longer-lasting effects than just the current cycle. Any time you artificially introduce hormonal substances, even naturally-occurring ones, into your body, it will take some time and patience to clear them even after you stop using them. So, if you have used birth control pills, injections, implanted birth control or the patch, your chances of getting pregnant right away may be somewhat compromised. There is a wide variety of anecdotal evidence that some women can get pregnant right away, even after using long-term birth control methods like Emplanon, an implant with a three-year effectiveness rating. There is an equal amount of anecdotal evidence that women taking the Pill have taken up to a year to conceive. How your body will react to birth control and stopping birth control is anybody's guess. The best advice we can give you is to wait until you are ready to conceive to stop taking your birth control method, but to be patient if conception doesn't happen right away.

If you have been trying for six months or a year without contraception, you may want to dig a little deeper for the reason. The quickest and probably cheapest way to do start your investigation is to invest in a basal temperature thermometer, also mentioned in the next section as a good early indicator that your period is late if you are irregular. With a basal temperature thermometer, you can chart your cycle, as your base temperature (upon awakening and before moving or getting out of bed) rises sharply just after ovulation. It is not, however, the best way to determine when to have intercourse for the best chance of conception, since you will want to time that for a couple of days before ovulation.

Nevertheless, once you are aware of the length of your cycle, you will have a better chance of timing it correctly. For the optimum results, try to have sex daily for the four or five days before you expect your ovulation, and on the same day. Do not worry about the old wives' tale that having sex too often can cause a low sperm count. If it is doing so, it is because there is an underlying condition that will have to be addressed to conceive anyway, and that will most likely be discovered later. Once you see that temperature spike, you can relax, and just watch for it to stay high beyond the expected start time for your period.

A higher-tech option is ovulation test strips, which purport to show you your most fertile two days. These work by detecting luteinizing hormone, which surges immediately before ovulation. Because viable sperm last in the Fallopian tubes much longer than an egg is viable, sex during the few days before ovulation is most likely to effect a meeting between sperm and egg. These test strips are fairly inexpensive; however, having a condition such as polycystic ovarian syndrome (which suppresses ovulation) can mean that you will need to use many test strips before detecting your optimum conception day. One woman reported ovulating on the 25th day of her cycle, as tested with these strips...a full 10 days beyond the normal ovulation cycle...and this was in the ninth month of attempting conception. If this option is one that interests you, you may also wish to know that there are a couple of different types, one used in mid-stream urination and another that is dipped into urine that you have captured in a container for the purpose. Choose the type that best suits your dexterity and budget.

What should you try next, if you determine that you are ovulating on a regular basis, and having sex during the optimum time, but you still have not been able to conceive within a reasonable time? It's time to investigate what could be going wrong with the other side of the equation. Before you even get to this point, be sure that dad is observing best practice, also. First, heat can have an adverse effect on sperm motility (the ability to swim to the objective) and viability (the strength to implant in the egg for fertilization). He should stop wearing briefs and switch to boxers for the time being, and should avoid hot tubs and saunas until you have conceived.

The next step is to have dad tested for low sperm count, low motility or viability. This is a difficult thing for most men to resort to, as it often makes them feel (inaccurately) less than virile. Try to understand if he is reluctant to see a doctor at first. If having a

21

baby is as important for him as it is for you, he will eventually realize that getting tested is perhaps the only way to solve the mystery of why you have not conceived. There are several solutions for these issues, so do not despair if the tests reveal that the problem is here. Consult your obstetrician for the best solution for your situation.

If nothing else seems to be wrong, it may just be a matter of patience. It goes without saying that everyone should stop smoking and using recreational drugs. By the way, once you have stopped, don't start again! But also look into the side effects of any prescription medications or supplements that either of you are taking. Additionally, any lubricant you might be using could have an adverse effect on sperm, so try to do without. Adopt a position for intercourse that will place the sperm in the optimal area for getting to the Fallopian tubes; i.e., avoid positions where they have to defy gravity. Finally, ask yourself whether stress might be playing a part. If the honest answer is yes, then the best thing you can do is try to relax, stop working at it so hard, and just let it happen naturally.

You think you're pregnant: what's next?

Signs and symptoms

Whether you have been trying to become pregnant or there are some signs and symptoms that make you think you may be, there are many reliable over-the-counter pregnancy tests that most women now use before contacting a doctor. Let's talk about what signs or symptoms might send you to a pharmacy to purchase a home pregnancy test.

Menstrual period late

If you have a regular menstrual cycle, the first sign that you may be pregnant is that you are late. You may not notice that for a while unless you have been trying; but sooner or later you will tumble to the fact that Mother Nature is late for your date. If your cycle is not regular, it may be several weeks before you notice. In fact, if your cycle is not regular, you may find it more difficult to conceive on request, so to speak. For irregular women, one way to help determine whether you are late is to acquire a basal temperature thermometer and keep a graph of your cycle. This special type of

23

thermometer can be obtained at pharmacies for about $15, and do not need a prescription.

There are many more detailed explanations of the whys and wherefores, both online and probably in the instructions that come with your thermometer, but the simple explanation is that your basal temperature (the temperature you can measure upon awakening and before getting out of bed or any other exertion) is slightly cooler before ovulation and slightly warmer after. We are talking about mere tenths of degrees, which is why you need a special thermometer for the accuracy. Although the Basal Body Temperature (BBT) is not a good predictor of ovulation— the fertile period—by charting your BBT you can get a sense of the body's rhythms and time intercourse to occur more often in the middle of the cycle, whenever that might be. But BBT is a great way to see an early indication that you might be pregnant. During a menstrual cycle that does not result in pregnancy, you will see a gradual drop in temperature after 7-10 days, followed by a steep drop on the day before you start your period. If you are pregnant, however, your BBT will remain high. If it has still not dropped within 18 days or more of ovulation, it's time to be tested.

OTC or home pregnancy tests range from about $10-25. We would recommend that you either ask your doctor for an opinion about which is most accurate, or perhaps look online for reviews of the tests. Home tests are generally considered accurate, assuming they are not expired and that you use them correctly and at the right time. They work by detecting the presence of hCG, a hormone that is only present when a woman is pregnant. However, levels of hCG are lower in the early days of a pregnancy, so if you take the test too early, you may get a false negative result. On the other hand, the only way to get a false positive is if you are taking a medication or a popular weight-loss supplement containing hCG. If you get a negative result from your home pregnancy test, keep taking your basal temperature. If it remains high and your period has still not shown up in a week or so, take another home test and see if you don't get a different result this time.

These simple methods will tell you whether or not you are pregnant some weeks before other symptoms of early pregnancy show up, and are relatively inexpensive. Once you have determined to your satisfaction that you are indeed pregnant, contact your doctor or midwife to set up your first appointment. It is important to receive qualified medical care throughout your pregnancy, to assure your baby's best chance at good health.

As your pregnancy progresses, you will likely experience other symptoms. Whether you will have all of the classic symptoms or only some depends on a lot of variables, and may be different from pregnancy to pregnancy even for the same woman. By the time some of them show up, you will have hopefully already seen the doctor for at least your first appointment. A few of them appear below, along with some tips for alleviating discomfort due to these symptoms. Before attempting any remedy you see here, be sure to check with your own doctor to be sure it is appropriate for your particular situation.

Morning sickness

Morning sickness' is nausea that can range from a mild queasy feeling upon smelling something that ordinarily would not bother you to severe, almost constant vomiting resulting in dehydration requiring medical intervention. No one really understands the causes of this nausea, which despite its name can occur any time during the day or night. Common theories are that hormonal changes such as raised levels of estrogen and progesterone and the introduction of hCG are to blame. Others blame a heightened sense of smell or disrupted digestive processes. More than likely, it is a combination of complex changes that your body requires time to adjust to. Although it is one of the most-recognized classic symptoms of pregnancy, it usually does not make an appearance until at least the sixth week after your last period.

Some tips include having a quick, easy to digest snack such as saltine crackers on hand, making sure that your stomach has something in it by spreading your food over several small meals per day, staying away from smells that seem to trigger your nausea, and doing your best to minimize stress. By all means, if you are still smoking, this should be a great incentive to quit, as smoke from cigarettes and cigars is a common trigger. It may help to jot down what you have been doing, smelling or eating just before experiencing an attack of nausea. By tracking what in particular might trigger your nausea, you are better armed to avoid it.

Some lucky women do not experience any nausea with pregnancy, while others can be miserable for months. If you are among the latter, rest assured that this will pass sooner or later. And the next pregnancy may give you a totally different experience, so think twice about vowing 'never again!' As a last resort, speak to your doctor about medication to control your nausea. Remember, however, that less medicine is best for your baby, and that not all medicines have received adequate testing to be sure they are safe.

If you can manage without medication, you will not regret that decision.

Fatigue

Fatigue, perhaps surprisingly, is one of the first symptoms to show up. Your body is on a tight schedule to prepare your baby's developmental environment. A flood of new or increased hormones has to be manufactured, and some of them are the same hormones that repair your muscles while you sleep. Having to pull double duty puts a lot of stress on your body. In addition, you are retaining some fluid for use in cushioning your tiny little one from the dangers of the outside world. You are gaining weight more rapidly than at any time since you were a baby yourself, and having to constantly re-adjust how your body is balanced is quietly taking its toll. No wonder you feel tired!

Some fatigue will be inevitable, but you can minimize its effects by, among other things, allowing yourself to be pampered. You may take on any and all challenges with an attitude that you are strong and can handle it, but just in this instance, drop the machismo and take all the help you can get. You and your growing babe deserve it! Take an afternoon nap if you can, but by all means get your full eight hours of sleep at night. Those hormones that are pulling double duty are manufactured during deep sleep, so make sure you get some.

That is not to say you should not continue your exercise routine, assuming you don't have an extreme one. You can and should both continue to eat nutritious food and get healthy exercise, although you may need to modify your exercise routine to keep your baby safe and you from being injured. We will explore exercise and nutrition both in later sections. Suffice it to say here that the better nutrition and the more consistent appropriate exercise you get, the less fatigue will be an issue for you.

It may be necessary to enlist the help of your spouse or partner, your parents, siblings, friends or even hire help to be able to get the rest you require. Do not let your pride stop you from asking for help. Most of your loved ones will be pleased to be a part of your pregnancy experience, and will be glad to help if you can let them know what help you need. Let someone else handle the heavy cleaning and laundry, you can return the favor another time.

Most women find that after the first three or four months, their energy returns and they feel great again until the very last few weeks before the birth. At this point, it is fine to do anything you feel like doing, with your doctor's approval. Avoid exertion that puts a strain on the muscles that support your growing abdomen, and anything that requires precise balance to avoid injury (like climbing ladders). This is the time to prepare a place in your home for baby's arrival. Talk to your doctor before painting, however. Many women experience the desire to clean their homes from top to bottom in preparation for the big event. Just be sensible about it. This is called the nesting instinct or phase, and often kicks in with a vengeance just a few weeks before baby's scheduled arrival, to be followed by extreme fatigue.

We are getting a bit ahead of ourselves here, but any discussion of fatigue symptoms would be incomplete if we did not mention that your fatigue is likely to return about the time your baby starts getting into birthing position. As baby turns and 'drops' toward the birth canal, your balance suddenly shifts again, the weight of baby and his internal environment pulls your back out of alignment and, if it has not happened previously, you can no longer walk without the distinctive waddle of advanced pregnancy. Get all the rest you can at this point, because it is soon to be a thing of the past!

Breast changes

Breast changes are to be expected, starting as early as the first trimester. Your body is preparing you for the important job of nourishing your baby, and even if you intend to bottle-feed, your body does not know it and will initiate the changes required for breastfeeding. Your breasts will certainly grow larger, and may become tender or easily irritated. By the fourth month of your pregnancy, you will probably notice leakage of fluid from your nipples, which have enlarged, darkened, and developed noticeable veins (due to increased blood supply) and bumps called Montgomery's tubercles around the areolae in the preceding months. The fluid is the early appearance of colostrum, a substance that is very important to your baby's early health, as it confers the mom's immunities to baby for a period of time and is packed with the nutrients that are perfect for the newborn until mom's milk comes in at around day 3 after your baby is born.

Those bumps around the nipple are important, too, as they signal production of an oily substance that keeps the skin moisturized and supple, as well as discouraging bacteria. Virtually all concerns that women have had regarding breastfeeding ever since we became 'civilized' and self-conscious about it are answered by the changes that your body knows to make all on its own!

Frequent urination

Frequent urination is another classic pregnancy symptom. Most pregnant women will start to notice urgency to go to the bathroom quite often, starting as early as six weeks into pregnancy. Part of the reason for this is because their kidneys are working extra hard to flush waste products from the increased blood supply from their bodies, placing a greater burden on the bladder. Of course part of that burden is also the pressure that is placed on the bladder by the growing uterus. Once baby starts to aim some well-placed kicks in that area, you could be in for some unwelcome surprises!

Abdominal cramping and pressure

One of the more disconcerting symptoms could be abdominal cramping and pressure. A woman usually becomes hypersensitive to any signals from the body that seem close in origin to where her baby is growing. The fact that there are plenty of other reasons for cramping and pressure than a pending problem for baby should ease your mind a bit. The most common cause is quite prosaic: bloating and gas caused by gastric disturbance related to your changing body and hormones or constipation. Toward the end of your pregnancy, you may experience Braxton-Hicks contractions, which are normal but do not signal the onset of labor. We'll discuss those in a different section.

If you experience severe or prolonged pain, bleeding or discharge, lower back pain or more than four hard contractions in an hour before close to your due date, it is a cause for real concern and you should contact your doctor immediately. Some causes for abdominal pain that are not necessarily related to your pregnancy but still require medical attention are food poisoning, bowel obstruction, kidney or gallbladder complications and fibroids. If in doubt, call your doctor and explain your symptoms.

Headaches

Some pregnant women complain of headaches when they were not subject to headache before, or an increase in headaches. The most likely causes of headaches during pregnancy are, once again, that old standby 'hormonal changes,' or blood sugar variations caused by changes in your body's response to food, whether that be nausea that prevents you from holding anything down or changes in your appetite. Do your best to avoid becoming dehydrated or excessively hungry to prevent headache. A surprising way to alleviate it is to drink something warm, and if your doctor has not recommended you cut out all caffeine, that could be a caffeinated beverage as caffeine also helps with this type of pain. If you are not allowed coffee or hot tea, think hot chocolate or even, if you can tolerate it, a glass of almost-hot water. Avoid heavy dependence on analgesics such as aspirin, ibuprofen or acetaminophen. Getting the appropriate amount of sleep can also ward off the tendency to get headaches, as stress and fatigue can contribute to them.

Mood swings

Mood swings are once again attributable to hormonal shifts or could be caused by your uncertainty about the unknown. Even expectant mothers who already have children can experience irrational fears about baby's health and safety, but for a new mom it is even worse: will you be able to handle labor and delivery (yes!), do you look fat (no, you look pregnant), are you as attractive to your spouse (most likely, but by all means talk about how you feel). Other concerns from financial stress to who will be insulted if the baby is not named after them seem to be much more intense when you are pregnant. Certainly how you feel physically can contribute to mood swings. Your best course of action is to talk with your loved ones and share your concerns, and do not worry if you are a bit snappish on occasion. After all, this is another classic symptom and most people will give you some leeway, assuming they know you are pregnant. If they don't, be ready with a charming apology, and maybe it is time to make that announcement!

Be sure to get plenty of rest, as lack of sleep can contribute, and as always, nutrition plays a huge part in how you feel.

Food cravings

Given half a chance, your grandmother would tell you that the foods you are craving are full of nutrients that your body is asking for. Some doctors would agree with her! However, if you are craving a tub of Rocky Road ice cream every night, you can be certain that it is more an emotional need you are trying to fill than a nutritional one. The best way to handle food cravings is to make a judgment about whether giving in to it will serve a nutritional need or whether it will sabotage your efforts to control your weight gain during pregnancy. If you are craving vegetables, go ahead and indulge. On the other hand, if it is something that is nutritionally empty and high in calories, try having just one or two bites, or distract yourself with something else until the craving goes away.

Remember that just because your condition is taking over your body, you are not required to let your mind follow. You can and should exercise the same control over unhealthy impulses now that you do when you are not pregnant; and all the more so if you have poor impulse control normally. Gaining too much weight while pregnant can lead to complications of the pregnancy that can threaten your unborn child with serious consequences.

Occasionally, you will experience an aversion to a food you normally enjoy. Unless the nutrients in it are available nowhere else, you do not have to force yourself to eat it. Doing so might even trigger the nausea reaction that is common during pregnancy. Other foods will have a strong odor that may offend your newly-sensitive olfactory processes, and you are welcome to avoid those as well. Chances are that your enjoyment of your favorite foods will return after your baby is born, so don't worry about it now—go ahead and avoid anything you don't want now until you want it again.

Finding your medical professionals

The care that women have been given during pregnancy has undergone amazing changes from the beginnings of time until now, and many of the changes have occurred during the past 30-50 years. Not long after World War II ended, almost all babies in the US were born in hospitals, with mom under anesthetic and under the care of a general practitioner. In the 1960s, a back-to-natural movement saw women insisting that they give birth at home, with midwives in attendance who may or may not have been medically trained. Nowadays, many women opt to be cared for by licensed nurse/midwives, who have received years of specialized medical training and who are overseen and backed up by OB/GYNs (obstetric and gynecologist) specialists in childbirth and women's health. Less often now, primarily because of malpractice lawsuits, a General Practitioner or Internal Medicine specialist may provide care during pregnancy and delivery. Because your primary care physician is likely one of the latter, if he does not accept pregnancy cases, he will usually refer you to an OB/GYN or nurse/midwife at your request. Whom you choose to care for you and deliver your baby is up to you, and here are some ideas to help you choose:

- Ask your primary care doctor for a referral
- Ask your friends
- Check with your insurance company to make sure they will pay whomever you choose

Ascertain whether your chosen medical professional is taking new patients and whether an appointment at the appropriate time is available; you might also want to find out if the doctor has an extended vacation or other away time scheduled during your pregnancy

Interview your final candidate to make sure you are a good fit. If not, keep looking until you find the person you will trust to care for you and your baby through delivery.

In addition to midwives, a recent addition to the team are trained labor coaches known as doulas. The assistance of a doula can shorten labor duration, reduce the need for medication, c-section and forceps, reduce health complications and hospitalization for baby as well as maternal hemorrhage, fever and infection after birth, and increase successful breastfeeding. Doulas educate and encourage new parents, assist with breathing and other considerations during labor, and make postpartum visits to ensure the health and welfare of mom and baby and to assist in any breastfeeding complications. Doula care has been shown to be superior to Lamaze and other natural-birth methodologies and promote the incidence of spontaneous vaginal birth, prompting some insurance companies to reimburse the expense.

Ideally, your first appointment should take place six to eight weeks after conception, unless there are other health concerns that you will need to address with your doctor. If you have chronic health problems like hypo- or hyper- thyroidism, chronic fatigue syndrome, fibromyalgia, diabetes or heart concerns, be sure to mention them to the person with whom you are scheduling the appointment. In these cases, you might need to be referred to a high-risk pregnancy specialist or at least be seen earlier rather than later for your first appointment.

What to expect at your first appointment

Of course your physician's office staff will go through the normal procedures that any doctor usually does, like taking your vital statistics, including weight, height, blood pressure, etc. They will almost certainly draw a blood sample and ask for a urine sample as well, to confirm the pregnancy among other things. You can expect the routine parts every time you have a doctor appointment.

During the first appointment either the doctor or his staff will take a detailed medical history. Be prepared to state the date of the first day of your last period, as this will give the doctor an idea of your due date to begin with. He will also want to know about previous pregnancies (if any), family/genetic concerns as far as you know them, your lifestyle including all those bad and good habits we have already discussed, and of course any chronic health concerns you have. He is highly likely to do a pelvic exam, and possibly an ultrasound exam. During this appointment, feel free to ask any questions or bring up any concerns you have about this pregnancy. Your doctor should be prepared to answer you in as much detail as you require—this will be a good test of whether you are a 'fit' for his doctor/patient relationship style.

You should be as emotionally comfortable with the physical exam as possible. Of course this is a very intimate exam, and if you are very young or inexperienced, it may be disconcerting. Keeping this in mind, pay attention to your feelings, and do not hesitate to look for another provider if you are more uncomfortable than you can explain. Many women find it helpful to select a female doctor. You have the right to have someone with you, either your spouse or a female relative, if it will help. As you progress through your pregnancy, you will probably be less emotionally uncomfortable with the proceedings. As far as physical comfort, well, that is to be desired but you may have to learn to endure a little indignity or discomfort. Just think about having a sweet little baby in your arms, and it won't be so bad after all.

At the first appointment, assuming you can state when your last period started, you may receive an estimated due date...but be aware that as your baby develops and more technology is brought to bear, that date may change. Your doctor will also make recommendations about diet, exercise and lifestyle changes if necessary, and will likely prescribe a prenatal vitamin containing special dosages of the vitamins and minerals that have been found to be most important to proper fetal development. These include folic acid and iron, in particular.

Future Appointments

For the next several months, your appointments will mostly be a matter of making sure you are (1) gaining the appropriate amount of weight, no more, no less; (2) your baby continues to exhibit the signs that are expected, like heartbeat, movement, etc. and (3) that you are having no unexpected symptoms or other health problems. We will cover what to expect in each trimester in a later section.

Healthy pregnancy lifestyle

The most obvious of changes during pregnancy concern weight gain. To help you understand why you will and must gain weight (except under highly unusual circumstances), here is a breakdown of what extra weight you will be carrying by the time you deliver your healthy baby:

- Baby: 7-8 pounds
- Placenta: 1-2 pounds
- Amniotic fluid: 2 pounds
- Uterus: 2 pounds
- Maternal breast tissue: 2 pounds
- Maternal blood : 4 pounds
- Fluids in maternal tissue: 4 pounds
- Maternal fat and nutrient stores: 7 pounds

Obviously, not everyone starts out at a healthy weight. How much you should expect to gain depends on your weight and BMI before pregnancy. BMI (Body Mass Index) is a rough indication of whether you are at a healthy weight as measured by fat ratio, calculated by a formula that takes into account your height vs. your weight. BMI is not a highly accurate measure of fat ratio, especially for athletes with a higher percentage of muscle mass (yes, including women) or someone who is much on either side of the average height. Still, it is one of the most common measurements of appropriate body composition. There are numerous online BMI calculators (just search under that term), some free, some associated with paid programs. The following list will give you an idea of how much weight you should gain in pregnancy according to your BMI.

- 25-35 pounds if you were a healthy weight before pregnancy (BMI of 18.5-24.9).
- 28-40 pounds if you were underweight before pregnancy (BMI of less than 18.5).
- 15-25 pounds if you were overweight before pregnancy (BMI of 25-29.9).
- 11-20 pounds if you were obese before pregnancy (BMI of over 30).

If you are carrying twins, consult with your doctor for appropriate weight gain. It will be more than the above, but not double. Multiples more than twins will also change the expectation.

This gain will be spread out over the course of your pregnancy, with 1-4.5 pounds being a good target for the first trimester and 1-2 pounds per week thereafter for a person who started out at a healthy weight. Extreme or prolonged morning sickness may keep you from gaining much during the first trimester, but should subside after the 20th week, at the longest. If you are over- or under-weight when you have your first appointment, your doctor will no doubt have some recommendations for you to help you with your baby's nutritional needs as well as your own.

It is important to gain the appropriate amount of weight at a steady pace during pregnancy as your developing little one requires daily nutrition from your diet just as you do. Dangers of being overweight or obese during your pregnancy include risk of gestational diabetes, discomfort such as backaches or leg pain, varicose veins and high blood pressure. Dangers of being underweight include low birth-weight baby (indicating malnourishment during gestation) and premature delivery. Your weight may fluctuate from week to week, and that is normal. However, a sudden gain or loss, especially in the third trimester, could mean complications and should be reported to your doctor immediately.

Nutrition

Having a healthy diet is always the best option, whether you are pregnant or not. Establishing healthy eating habits and making sure you are at a healthy weight before you become pregnant is the best course of action, as we mentioned in the beginning sections of this book. Doing so without the added stressors of pregnancy and without the cravings and food aversions is far easier than doing so with all those extra considerations. Whether or not you had that luxury, now that your pregnancy has been confirmed, it is essential for a number of reasons, not the least of which is ensuring that your baby has all the nutrients she needs to grow strong and healthy for her birth.

Assuming you were at an appropriate weight before pregnancy, neither overweight nor underweight, you will need to slowly increase your calorie intake to meet the needs of your growing baby. By your second trimester, you should be consuming an extra 300 calories per day and by the third, an extra 450. However, please do not use this as a license to load up on junk food! Larger portions of your healthy choices, or more portions spread throughout the day is the way to increase your calories responsibly. There are many guides, including the simple 'plate' graphic that has replaced the old USDA 'food pyramid,' to help you choose what foods to eat and in what proportions. Here are a few of the highlights:

Macronutrients

Macronutrients are the three major types of food, that is, protein, carbohydrates and fat. Within these foods are micronutrients, i.e., vitamins, minerals, bioflavonoids, etc. To begin to construct a healthy diet, you should make sure your ratios of the macronutrients are appropriate for your condition. Most doctors do not recommend a weight-loss regimen while you are pregnant, because weight-reduction diets typically skew certain nutrients out of proportion, so we will talk about the ratios for an average, healthy 150-lb. woman who is moderately active throughout pregnancy. Consult your doctor or a nutritionist if you were over- or under-weight when you became pregnant or if you are considerably shorter or taller than the average, to determine your dietary requirements.

A simple way to determine your basic calorie needs is to multiply your weight by 12 if you are moderately active, or by 10 if you are more sedentary. Therefore, to maintain her weight, a woman who weighs 150 lbs. should consume between 1500 and 1800 calories per day. This of course assumes that 150 lbs. is your appropriate weight, but it serves as a good starting point for the average woman. Of that amount of calories, 45-65% should come from carbohydrates, or, for the 1800-calorie basis, 810-1170 should come from carbohydrates. Furthermore, most of those should be in the form of fiber; in other words, the bulk of your diet should be made up of whole grains and starchy vegetables. Because this flies in the face of modern weight-loss theory and does not take into account the sensitivity to gluten that many modern women experience, you should attempt to balance this dietary need with your overall dietary concerns as well as your doctor's recommendations.

Recommendations for the next-highest ratio macronutrient, surprisingly, is fat. By this we mean healthy fats, which should comprise between 20 and 35% of your daily calorie intake, or between 360 and 630 calories per day. Within this ratio are also saturated and trans-fats, which are sometimes unavoidable but are not desirable. Saturated fat should comprise less than 10% of your calories per day, while you should avoid trans-fat altogether if possible. Healthy fats come from nuts, seeds, fruits like avocado and oils that are liquid at room temperature, such as olive oil and other vegetable oils. Saturated fats are usually found in animal products—meat, whole milk and butter, for example. Trans-fats are usually found in junk foods, and can be identified by the words 'hydrogenated' or 'partially hydrogenated' in the list of ingredients. If you are overweight, do not be tempted to skimp on the healthy fats while you are pregnant, as it could have serious consequences for your baby's development.

Finally, protein is recommended to be between 10 and 35 percent of your daily calories. Remember that protein is found in many foods other than meat, eggs and dairy products. The lowly Idaho potato contains 7.5 grams of protein for a medium-sized one, for example.

Five food groups

Lest you despair about counting all these calories and proportions, another way of looking at it is to get the proper variety from the five food groups (which both roughly correspond to and overlap the three macronutrients.) For a healthy adult woman, three servings of protein, two servings of fruit, five servings of vegetables, six servings of grain and 2-3 servings of dairy. Don't worry if you are confused about all this—many adults are, as it is not a universal part of our educational system. There are many online resources and chances are your doctor has a brochure or pamphlet she can give you to help you make good choices. Meanwhile, make sure those vegetable and fruit choices include a good variety of both, eat sweets and junk food in moderation if at all, and make sure the cereals and grains you consume are whole grain, and you should be fine.

Other nutritional considerations

Pay particular attention to including the following nutrients in greater proportions in your pregnancy diet:

Iron is needed in greater supply both for baby's developing blood supply and for mom's, which doubles during this time. Most pre-natal supplements contain some, but you may need a second supplement in addition to what you can get from red meat, deep green leafy vegetables and cooked legumes as well as sardines and soy products if you can tolerate them.

Calcium is essential to protect mom's bone density during pregnancy. Your baby will take what he needs as he develops, and if you are not consuming enough, it will come from your bones. You need a minimum of 1200 milligrams a day, which is difficult to get from food sources. Milk and other dairy products, calcium-fortified orange juice, sardines, broccoli and green leafy vegetables such as spinach have high levels of calcium, but you would have to consume far more than a normal person could to get the amount of calcium needed during pregnancy. Therefore, follow your doctor's recommendation for a supplement. There is much debate on what form of calcium is most readily absorbed into your body, but all forms have improved bioavailability if taken with Vitamin D.

Fluids are more important now than ever. An appropriate intake of water and other fluids will help to flush toxins from your body, prevent constipation and hydrate your skin, hair and nails from the inside, always. While you are pregnant, it will also promote healthy development of your baby's kidneys and liver and promote a good milk supply.

3 Very important tips

- Eat breakfast every day
- Snack between meals to keep blood sugar level and avoid nausea
- Be sure to get sufficient protein

Supplements

It is highly likely that your doctor will prescribe a prenatal vitamin, formulated especially to supply adequate folic acid and Vitamin D. Lack of the former has been implicated in various neural tube defects, including spina bifida, so medical research has determined that an added amount over and above the recommended daily allowance for most adults is the best way to avoid these defects. Some doctors will prescribe a prenatal formula even before you become pregnant if they are aware that you are trying or intend to try. This is the only supplement needed by most healthy women, but several others may be prescribed if you have some health problems, which we will cover in a later section.

Do not take supplements that are not formulated for pregnant women, including extra herbal, vitamin or mineral supplements, without your doctor's approval. Some herbal substances interfere with the action of vitamins and minerals, others interfere with prescribed medications, and there is always the risk of getting too much of a good thing. Even if your doctor approves, it would not hurt to also consult your pharmacist, who may know more about what interacts with what than even a doctor.

Now is not the time to decide to improve your memory with ginkgo biloba, or lose weight with whatever the latest herbal remedy is, so avoid anything that you do not absolutely need, and check with professionals before you even take that. By the way, that advice also goes for over-the-counter medication, such as aspirin, ibuprofen, etc. Ask before you take it!

Foods to avoid

In general, you will want to avoid junk foods and other foods high in unhealthy fats and salt, just as you would in everyday life. However, there are a few foods that are perfectly fine for a healthy adult but are on the off-limits list for your developing baby.

Seafood

Yes, fish is a very healthy protein and you should probably eat more than most people do. However, avoid raw or undercooked seafood and especially raw shellfish like oysters and clams. Stay away also from certain fish known to be high in mercury, as mercury contamination can interfere with your baby's developing nervous system. These include tilefish, king mackerel, shark and swordfish.

Unpasteurized dairy

Although most milk today is pasteurized, it is still possible to get unpasteurized milk from sources that are not produced for the mass market. If you buy your milk from the local dairy, make sure it is pasteurized and that they are complying with all health and safety regulations. Some cheeses are unpasteurized by definition, including Camembert, Brie and Blue Cheese, as well as other unpasteurized soft cheeses.

Undercooked and improperly handled foods

Undercooked meat, eggs or poultry could cause bacterial contamination, as can improperly refrigerated foods. If you have ever had food poisoning, you know what havoc it can wreak on an adult body. How much more devastating do you think it would be for your unborn baby? Err on the side of caution when deciding whether to eat that Thanksgiving turkey or Fourth of July potato salad that has been sitting out all day, or that rare hamburger patty. Even if someone else in the family has eaten some without ill effect, you should avoid the risk.

Be sure that any food you intend to consume raw, such as fruits or vegetables, have been thoroughly washed and if cut, have been cut with clean implements. Harmful pesticides or human contamination by handlers, from those who pick the produce to those who stack it in your local grocer's shelves, can remain on unwashed produce. Bacterial contamination from something else cut with that knife could be introduced if you don't wash it before using it to cut food you will eat raw.

Caffeine

Some doctors prefer that you avoid caffeine altogether, others want you to limit it to perhaps no more than 200 milligrams per day. A regular cup of coffee might contain about 95 mg. Tea contains less. Caffeine has been shown to have the effect of raising fetal heart rate, which is not considered a good thing. Note that many popular soft drinks as well as hot chocolate have some caffeine also.

Alcohol

It bears repeating that it is best to avoid alcohol in any amount, for reasons we have already stated.

Exercise and Other Activity

Your exercise program

Not only for weight control, but also because an active mom can expect fewer negative symptoms of pregnancy and a more comfortable delivery, it is important to exercise. If you have been active before becoming pregnant, you can usually continue your exercise or recreational routine. However, if your routine includes activities with a high risk of falling or other jarring impact, do consult with your doctor. Chances are your own comfort will lead you to modify your routine if it includes aerobics with a lot of high-impact work. One thing you can and should do is walk at a pace that is as brisk as you can manage. Aim for at least three 30-minute exercise sessions per week, just as if you were not pregnant. If you can manage more, so much the better.

If you have been sedentary, and especially if you are very overweight, it is better to start out more slowly, and always consult your physician before beginning an exercise program. A good rule of thumb is to exercise more consistently even if that means you can't do much at a time. Maybe all you can do to begin is walk to your mailbox and back. That's fine...but do it two or three times a day until you can go farther. By the time your baby is born, maybe you'll be able to push the stroller all the way around the nearest park—won't that be wonderful?

It is not necessary to go to a gym and sweat to have an effective workout. Of course, if that is your preference, go right ahead within the limits that your physician and your own body set for you. If not, take comfort in the fact that studies have shown three ten-minute cardio sessions spread out over the course of a day to be as effective as one half-hour all at once. The bottom line here is to not overdo it. There is no need to push yourself to the point of exhaustion, and in fact that will be counterproductive.

Remember to warm up, cool down, and stretch gently. These are necessary steps in a proper exercise program that will protect you from injury as you work out. Stretching after warm up prevents injury, and after cool down it both prevents muscular soreness and feels wonderful! Never push your stretch beyond what is comfortable, as that is a sure way to injure yourself.

One special exercise does not require great effort but will greatly assist in your labor when the time comes. Known as a Kegel exercise, it consists of repeatedly contracting and relaxing the muscles of the pelvic floor. It requires no special equipment, and can be done anywhere and at any time, even while doing other things! To perform a Kegel exercise, simply contract your pelvic floor muscles as if you were stopping the flow of urine, hold for a few seconds, and then relax. Repeat several times, as often as you remember. This exercise is reported to have many benefits besides those for pregnancy, including treating urinary incontinence and increasing sexual gratification.

Working while pregnant

What about working? The same advice goes. If you can be safe physically and your job does not require exertion that puts strain on your growing abdomen, you should be able to work as long as you wish to. Recently it has become common for women to work right up until they feel the first contraction or until their water breaks. On the other hand, if your work is dangerous or exposes you and your unborn baby to unusual environmental hazards, it would be best to either ask for a transfer to a safer area or take leave until baby is safely born.

Your employer is legally required to make accommodations for a temporary condition like pregnancy, so do not worry about losing your job if you must modify it because of your pregnancy. Do get a note from your doctor to back you up on the request. If you experience discrimination because of your pregnancy, your HR department or state agency that controls fair labor practices will assist you.

Of course, if you prefer not to work, intend to stay at home with your baby rather than returning to work, and have the luxury of the choice, there is no reason you should not quit working as soon as you wish. Do note that your work-related health insurance will not automatically pay for the rest of the pregnancy and delivery if you have left your job. If you are dependent on your own health insurance, check before you make any irrevocable decisions. You may be able to continue your insurance for a period of time after you resign.

Everyday activities

Use common sense when it comes to every day activity such as recreational pursuits (you should probably stop skydiving, for example) and even common household activities. If it hurts to mop the floor, enlist your spouse or a friend to help with that chore. Avoid getting on ladders or high step-stools, as your balance is affected as your body grows. Avoid the use of household chemicals that might be dangerous if inhaled or mixed with other chemicals.

Avoid hot tubs, saunas and steam rooms, as you should not expose your baby to body temperatures over 102°F for extended periods. Swimming is not only fine but encouraged, as it is good exercise with no impact to jar your body. Just use common sense about the temperatures involved as well as where you swim (i.e., better to avoid the river downstream from that chemical plant.)

There are a few myths, or old wives tales if you prefer, about what you should and shouldn't do while pregnant. One that seems to make a little sense at first glance and needlessly worries many women is that if you lift your arms above your head it will cause your baby's umbilical cord to become tangled or wrapped around her neck. This is absolutely not true, so go ahead and put the dishes away or hang your sheets on an outdoor clothesline...it will not harm your baby. When such unfortunate occurrences happen, it is because of fetal movement, not mom's.

One thing you should stop doing at all until after your baby is born is cleaning the cat box. Cat litter can be infected by a parasitic disease called toxoplasmosis, which can be transmitted to the fetus if mom becomes newly infected while pregnant.

Toxoplasmosis is a leading cause of death due to food borne illness and is considered a neglected parasitic disease by the Centers for

Disease Control because not much attention is paid to it other than warning pregnant women not to clean cat boxes. It is thought that more than 60 million men, women and children in the US are infected by the parasite, which usually causes no symptoms in a healthy individual because the immune system keeps it under control. However, as you can see, it is very dangerous to a developing fetus or a person with a compromised immune system. Less often mentioned, but still something to consider, is whether you should be gardening if there are many neighborhood cats ranging freely outside—your flowerbeds could be de facto cat boxes. If you cannot avoid either of these activities, wear a face mask and heavy protective gloves while doing them.

Sex during pregnancy

You may or may not feel like it, but sex during pregnancy is just fine, again except under highly unusual circumstances. Many women find that their libido is greater, possibly because they no longer have to fear becoming pregnant, or possibly because the increased hormones flooding their bodies contribute to a feeling of relaxation and well-being. Many men find their partners' changing bodies extremely attractive and desirable, and their appreciation may make their partners feel more open to enjoying sexual relations. There is no physical reason not to indulge, although there may come a time during your pregnancy that adjustments in position are required. If you feel your baby is not arriving on schedule, some doctors will even mention having sex as a possible remedy for the situation, so even late in pregnancy, sex is okay. However, once your mucous plug has dislodged or your water has broken, avoid sex as it may introduce bacteria to the birth canal.

Healthy meals during pregnancy

Below are a few recipes from my book – **Pregnancy Nutrition** – that contains more than 60 healthy and nutritious recipes for breakfast, lunch, dinner and desserts. You can find the book on my Amazon author page here http://amazon.com/author/john-mcarthur

3 Easy breakfast recipes

Fresh Herb Omelet

Ingredients

3 free-range eggs

1/2 tsp extra virgin olive oil

2 tbsp finely shredded fresh herbs: Parsley, basil, chives, parsley, and marjoram

Salt and Pepper

1 tsp unsalted butter

Wholewheat bread

Preparation

In a medium sized bowl, whisk the eggs and season with salt and pepper.

Heat the butter and oil in a frying pan. Once it starts to sizzle, pour in the egg mixture. As the bottom of the omelet starts to cook, lift it on one side and allow the uncooked egg to run underneath it.

Keep doing this until the omelet is cooked all the way through.

Top one side of the cooked omelet with the shredded herbs and fold over. Carefully remove the omelet from the pan and plate. Serve with toasted Wholewheat bread.

Guilt-Free Breakfast Pizza

Ingredients

1 whole wheat thin pizza base

¼ cup cheese

2 tbs pizza sauce

1 tbsp of chopped green pepper

1 tbsp fresh basil

Preparation

Spread the pizza sauce on the base and then add the basil, cheese, green pepper, and basil.

Place in the microwave for 1 min until the cheese has melted.

Delicious Oats topped with Bananas and Walnuts

Ingredients

1 1/3 cup rolled oats

2 cups water

1 cup low-fat milk

2 thickly sliced medium sized bananas

1/2 cup chopped walnuts

1 tbsp honey

1 additional cup low-fat milk (for use on cooked oats – optional)

Preparation

Pour the water and the milk (1 cup) into a pot and bring to the boil.

Lower the heat and add oats. Allow to simmer for about 5 min.

Oats should be soft and creamy when ready.

Put oats in bowls and top with honey, walnuts and banana sliced.

Add extra milk if desired. Serves 4.

Healthy dinner recipes

Curry Infused Beef Pilaf

Ingredients

14 oz (400g) lean beef mince

1 1/2 tbsp olive oil

3 finely chopped green onions

8.8 oz (250g) cherry tomatoes

1 cup rinsed basmati rice

2 1/2 cups chicken stock (reduced salt)

1 tbsp curry powder

1/2 cup flat-leaf parsley leaves

1 tsp ground cumin

1 tsp ground cinnamon

1/4 cup currants

Preparation

Preheat oven to 365°F (180°C). Now lay cherry tomatoes on a baking tray on some baking paper. Pour 2 teaspoons of oil over the tomatoes and season with salt and pepper. Place in oven for 20 minutes until tomatoes become soft.

Place a saucepan on the stove on medium heat and add remaining oil. Add the cumin, cinnamon, curry powder and mince to heated oil and allow to cook while stirring for 4 minutes. Add rice.

Pour the chicken stock into the rice dish and bring to the boil. Now pour the mixture into a large oven dish. Cover and bake for approximately 25 minutes, or until all the liquid has been soaked into the rice.

To add the finishing touches, stir the tomatoes, currants and green onions into the dish. Allow to stand for a few minutes before serving. Add parsley just before dishing up. Serves 4

Chicken and Sun-dried Tomato Pasta

Ingredients

10.6 oz (300g) chicken breast fillet slices

14.10 oz (400g) fettuccine pasta

2 tsp olive oil

12.7 fl. oz. (375ml) evaporated milk

1.7 oz (50g) baby spinach

2 shredded green onions

1/2 cup chopped sun-dried tomatoes

1/4 cup pitted black olives

1 tbsp corn flour

Wholewheat Bread

Preparation

Cook pasta according to package directions until al Dente. Once cooked, drain and place back into the pot that you cooked it in.

While the pasta is cooking, heat some oil in a pan. Fry onions until brown before adding chicken pieces. Continue to cook for another

3 minutes or until chicken is cooked the way you like it. Now add the black olives and tomatoes. Toss.

In a jug combine the corn flour with 1 tbsp of cold water and stir to form a paste before stirring in the evaporated milk.

Pour the mixture over the chicken in the frying pan and allow to cook for 2 minutes until the sauce thickens. Season as desired.

Add the contents of the frying pan to the cooked pasta and toss in the baby spinach. Allow to cook over low heat for a few minutes.

Serve with buttered whole-wheat bread. Serves 4.

Spicy grilled Fish and Fresh Vegetables

Ingredients

4 x (5.30 oz or 150g each) firm white fish fillets

2 tbsp olive oil

1 tsp smoked paprika

1 1/3 cups flat-leaf parsley leaves

Juice from 1/2 lemon

2 thinly diced zucchini

2 baby eggplants, sliced diagonally

1 halved and chopped red capsicum

5 ¼ oz (150g) diced button mushrooms

Crispy wholewheat bread

Preparation

Drizzle some olive oil into a large pan and heat on medium high heat. While you wait, season the fish with oil and paprika. Place the zucchini, capsicum, mushrooms and eggplant in bowl and coat with 1 tbsp of oil. Season the vegetables to taste with salt and pepper.

Cook the vegetables on a heated barbeque plate for 8 to 10 minutes whilst turning. Once they have browned, place them in a bowl and toss with parsley and 1 1/2 tbsp of lemon juice.

Cook the seasoned fish on the same grill for 2 minutes per side and then serve with wholewheat bread and golden brown vegetables. Serves 4.

3 Quick and healthy lunch recipes

Delicious Chicken Tortilla

Ingredients

1 sliced chicken breast

1 tsp olive oil

1 finely chopped onion

1roughly chopped red or green pepper

A few small tortillas

1 peeled and grated carrot

1 cup of lettuce

14 oz. drained kidney beans

1 tbsp crème fraiche

Salt and pepper

Preparation

Fry the onion and pepper in the tsp of olive oil for approximately 2 minutes.

Add the chicken pieces and continue frying until the chicken is cooked and nicely browned.

In a separate bowl combine and crème fraiche and kidney beans and mash.

Spread the mixture onto a few tortillas and then add the chicken, lettuce leaves and carrots before you roll it up. Guaranteed to be delicious!

Turkey and Coleslaw Sandwich

Ingredients

2 cups grated carrot and cabbage (mixed)

2 tbsp low fat Italian salad dressing

2 slices of rye bread

9 oz. thinly slices turkey breast (cooked)

3 slices provolone cheese

1 thinly sliced tomato

Cucumber slices

Preparation

Place coleslaw mix in a bowl and combine with Italian dressing.

Place rye bread slices on a plate and top with turkey, cheese slices, tomato slices, coleslaw, and cucumber slices.

Close sandwich and toast in a heated pan – 4 min per side or until cheese is melted.

Vegetarian Open Sandwich

Ingredients

2 tsp Dijon mustard

1/4 cup grated carrot

1/2 cup broccoli florets (small)

2 toasted whole-wheat English Muffins

1/4 cup roughly chopped red bell pepper

1/2 cup shredded Monterey Jack Cheese (Low Fat)

Preparation

Turn on oven (grill)

Spread Dijon mustard over all sides of English muffin and top with broccoli, carrots and bell peppers. Finish of with shredded cheese.

Place under grill for a few min, or until cheese has melted.

Sweet and healthy

Refreshing Vanilla Yoghurt and Mango Pops

Ingredients

3 chopped up ripe mangoes

260g (1 cup) low fat vanilla yoghurt

Preparation

Place the mangoes into a food processor and blend until smooth. Remove the mango puree and combine with the vanilla yoghurt in a separate bowl.

Transfer the vanilla and mango mixture into an ice tray that has at least 8 80 ml sections. Place the tray in the freezer and leave to freeze for at least 8 hours. Refreshing and delicious!

Pecan, Almond and Dried Fruit Bars

Ingredients

45g (1/3 cup) roughly chopped pecan nuts

60g (1/3 cup) chopped blanched almonds

25g (1/3 cup) diced dried apples

70g (1/3 cup) diced dried apricots

90g (1 cup) rolled oats

1 tbsp light olive oil

2 tbsp maple syrup

Preparation

Preheat oven to 180°C. In a medium bowl combine the rolled oats with the olive oil and maple syrup. Scatter the oats onto a baking tray and bake in the preheated oven for 5 minutes. Remove from the oven and scatter the almonds and pecans over the oat mixture. Stir to combine and then place back into the oven for 6 more minutes. The nuts should be brown and crispy once they are done.

Remove the oat mixture from the oven and transfer the contents into a large bowl. Now add the dried fruit and mix.

Store the bars in an airtight container. Sprinkle the bars over tinned fruit, yoghurt, or cereal.

Mixed Berry and Banana Smoothie

Ingredients

1/2 cup low-fat milk

1/2 cup low-fat vanilla yoghurt

4 ice cubes

1 large sliced banana

2 tsp honey

1/2 cup mixed berries

2 teaspoons wheat germ

Preparation

Place all the ingredients in a blender and blend until smooth.
Serves 2.

Common health issues during pregnancy

It goes without saying that a chronic health condition or disease might spell trouble for your unborn baby from the word go. Nevertheless, many women who have the following conditions are able to deliver healthy babies with proper medication and healthcare support, so do not despair that you will not be able to bear children if you have them. If you are chronically ill, it would probably be best to speak to your primary care physician and possibly a high-risk pregnancy specialist before becoming pregnant. Here are some things to consider for each condition.

Anemia

There are three types of anemia: iron-deficiency, folate deficiency, and B12 deficiency. Risks of severe anemia of any type include delivering a low birth-weight or preterm baby, need for transfusion if severe bleeding occurs, and for the folate or B12 deficiency, risk of neural tube defects (birth defects involving the spine or brain).

The most common cause of anemia is lack of one of these nutrients in the diet. A mom with a poor diet or, in some cases, vegetarian or vegan diet may not get enough of these nutrients, all of which are found in meat as the richest source. Supplementing the diet with iron and folate in pill or tablet form or B12 in the form of injections, is called for. Vegans should be tested for B12 and receive injections as required whether pregnant or not, as it is not possible to obtain this nutrient in sufficient quantities as a vegan, no matter how healthy your choices are.

Your physician will usually test for anemia at your first appointment and one or more times throughout your pregnancy, but definitely call her attention to the following symptoms if you experience them:

- Pale skin, lips, and nails
- Feeling tired or weak
- Dizziness
- Shortness of breath
- Rapid heartbeat
- Trouble concentrating

All pregnant women are at risk for becoming anemic during pregnancy, due to the increased demands the baby makes on your body and in some cases because of nausea contributing to insufficient nutrient absorption. At increased risk are teenagers, women whose periods were abnormally heavy before pregnancy, moms pregnant with more than one child or having two or more pregnancies close together, in addition to those who experience severe morning sickness or whose diets do not support nutritional adequacy of iron, folate or B12.

To avoid anemia during pregnancy, include more of the following iron-rich foods in your diet:

- lean red meat, poultry, and fish
- leafy, dark green vegetables (such as spinach, broccoli, and kale)
- iron-enriched cereals and grains
- beans, lentils, and tofu
- nuts and seeds
- eggs

To help absorb the iron, add the following foods high in Vitamin C at the same meals:

- citrus fruits and juices
- strawberries
- kiwis
- tomatoes
- bell peppers

Some of the preceding lists are also high in folates, but to get even more, choose fortified breads and cereals to add to your daily diet.

Autoimmune disorders

Pregnancy may or may not have an effect on an existing autoimmune disorder, and if it does, the effect might be good rather than bad. However, because autoimmune disorders are not well-understood, it is likely that your primary care physician will not be able to advise you on your specific situation. Consult a specialist in the disorder or a high-risk pregnancy specialist to determine whether a pregnancy is advisable, or to monitor your situation if you are already pregnant and have a preexisting autoimmune disorder, or if you develop one during pregnancy (example, autoimmune thyroiditis).

Depression

Post-partum depression is rather common, but what if you begin to experience depression during pregnancy, or have clinical depression before becoming pregnant? Because clinical depression is a brain-chemistry issue, and brain chemistry means hormones, this is not uncommon either, but there is a reason to talk to your doctor about it. If you are depressed during pregnancy, it may be difficult for you to bond with your child after delivery. This is a tragic consequence, leading to far-reaching developmental, mental and social consequences for your baby. If you have never known anyone with clinical depression, you may not understand why you are tearful, anxious, sad or moody nor realize that these normal transient symptoms of pregnancy are exaggerated in your case. Pay attention if your friends or loved ones exhibit concern for these symptoms, and ask your doctor. It is treatable, so do not ignore it and hope it will go away.

Diabetes

Pregnancy in a mom who has diabetes is considered high-risk. If you have diabetes, you should consult a doctor specializing in high-risk pregnancies before becoming pregnant. If you are not diabetic, but have a family history of diabetes or are seriously overweight, you are at increased risk of gestational diabetes, which is a temporary condition associated with your pregnancy. The fact that it is temporary, however, does not mean that it is of no concern. Far-reaching consequences for the baby, beginning with high birth weight and attendant complications of possible c-section should be enough to help you realize you must keep this under control. Being overweight can raise mom's blood pressure, leading to pre-eclampsia or eclampsia, a serious condition that can cause fetal death. It is essential to control weight gain whether or not you are at higher risk for diabetes or gestational diabetes.

Thyroiditis

Thyroiditis can present as either underactive or over active thyroid, and can be autoimmune in nature or not.

Your baby requires an adequate level of thyroid hormone for proper brain and nervous system development. If you had hypothyroidism (underactive thyroid gland) before pregnancy, your medication level may have to be adjusted throughout your pregnancy to keep up with increased demand. If you were not already experiencing hypothyroidism, but develop severe fatigue, a lump in your throat near the voice box, begin to lose your hair or experience out-of-control weight gain, you may ask your doctor if you need to be tested. It is possible to have a low-functioning thyroid gland without experiencing symptoms until pregnancy throws you into frank hypothyroidism. Because the consequences for baby are so serious, including low IQ, it is important to stay on top of this one.

Hyperthyroidism can lead to low birth weight, pre-term delivery and neonatal hyperthyroidism, which if left untreated can lead to death. Symptoms of hyperthyroidism are nervousness and anxiety, goiter, inability to gain weight and heart palpitations. Like its opposite, it is possible to have a subclinical case before pregnancy that is exacerbated by the pregnancy itself.

Other complaints

Obviously we cannot provide an exhaustive list of chronic illnesses and describe their effects on pregnancy and vice versa. Those we have explored are relatively common, but there are many more that we have not explored. It bears repeating that if you are uncertain about your health you would be well-advised to seek medical opinion before attempting to conceive. If after you conceive you develop signs and symptoms that are not mentioned here or elsewhere as common to pregnancy, bring them up with your doctor so that they can be addressed before adversely affecting your own long-term health or your baby's development.

Sleeping position and stillbirth

Something no expectant mother wants to face and may refuse to think about in a superstitious dread that thinking about it will make it happen, is that a developing fetus is highly vulnerable to so many things beyond our control. The list of maternal illnesses in the previous section may have already sent terror into your heart and mind, and that was not our intention. To the extent possible, we want you to be aware of your own health and those things that you can be in control of, to give your baby the best chance possible of being born healthy and staying that way.

One of the most surprising things that have come out of medical research in the past few years is that maternal sleeping position has a profound effect on baby's chances of survival. Your doctor may or may not be aware of studies linking a higher incidence of stillbirth to mom's sleeping position; specifically, sleeping on the back. Fortunately, Nature herself takes care of that as sleeping on back or stomach becomes more and more uncomfortable as your baby grows. Nevertheless, we must take this opportunity to highly recommend you sleep on your side, preferably the left side.

Sleeping on your side makes it easier for your heart to do its job without the weight of the fetus restricting the large vein (inferior vena cava) that carries your blood back from your lower extremities to your heart. Naturally, that also helps your baby's oxygenation. In addition, sleeping on the left side keeps the baby off the liver, another large organ whose function is both critical to baby's health and is subjected to more stress during the pregnancy.

To achieve the most comfort in the recommended position, try experimenting with pillows behind your back, under your abdomen or between your knees or ankles. Body-length pillows might make it even easier to find the position in which you are most comfortable. Look also for specifically-designed pregnancy pillows that prevent you from rolling onto your back or stomach.

An added benefit to sleeping on your side is relief from lower-back pain that can occur as your body shifts to accommodate the increased weight in front, as well as lessening the incidence of heartburn that could become an issue during pregnancy.

The stages of pregnancy

Although a full-term pregnancy, including the approximately two weeks between the beginning of your last period and conception, is closer to 40 weeks than the traditional nine months, we still describe the stages of pregnancy in terms of trimesters, or thirds, of approximately three months each, with an extra week thrown in here and there.

Before the days of accurate determination of date of conception, doctors had to rely on what could be very subjective observations from external exams, measuring the growth of your abdomen or the like to determine due date. This resulted in some humorous errors, for example in the case of the woman carrying twins whose basal temperature record indicated a due date in late February, while the doctor's measurements kept advancing due date until it had her five weeks overdue in mid-January. The fact that ultrasound has also only been commonplace in the last two decades made it more likely for this type of error. If the baby was much larger or smaller than average, a multiple birth had not been suspected for some reason, or mom did not keep an accurate record of her menstrual cycle, expectant mothers might find themselves racing for the hospital unexpectedly!

Now, of course, anyone with access to modern medicine should have a very good idea of the progress of her baby's development, and a somewhat accurate estimate of due date. Of course, Mother Nature is not a Swiss clock, so there is still some room for error. Here are the broad strokes of what you can expect in each trimester.

First trimester—weeks 1 to 12

Doctors use the beginning of your last period to start this weekly count, so strictly speaking you are not really pregnant until your ovulation has occurred and the ovum has been fertilized, at the end of about week two. Your first inkling may be that your period is late after two more weeks (or so) or that your basal temperature has not dropped at that time indicating that your period is about to start. If you have been trying to conceive, the next few days might be the most stressful of your entire pregnancy, as you anxiously watch for signs that your hopes are to be dashed. After a week or so, your anxiety might tempt you to obtain a home pregnancy test. The longer you can wait to give in to this temptation, the more accurate your test results will be, but remember that it is unlikely that you will get a false positive. As the excitement builds, you will no doubt succumb to temptation and at some point will see that positive indicator that means you are definitely pregnant.

As the next few weeks unfold, you will contact your preferred medical professional to take care of you and your baby during your pregnancy, ideally scheduling your first appointment for about the sixth week. Whether you confine your good news to your spouse or a few close friends and family members or announce it to the world likely has to do with your personality and how many times you have announced prematurely. Between the sixth and eighth week, however, your body may provide a hint by sending you often to the ladies room with morning sickness, or filling out your bras more noticeably.

This trimester may feel more like three years, between keeping the secret (if you do) and the physical discomforts that are making themselves known. Meanwhile, your baby is making the most of it, miraculously developing from one fertilized ovum into a tiny, perfectly formed little human about three inches long. By eight weeks, he is moving a lot, but you aren't likely to be able to feel it for some time to come unless this is not your first pregnancy. By the end of twelve weeks, your baby's organs, limbs and features, right down to hair follicles and fingernails, have started to develop. Odds of miscarriage drop dramatically by this point in the timeline.

Second trimester—weeks 13 to 29

As you move into the second trimester, you may find that some of the more uncomfortable symptoms of pregnancy have either subsided or you are becoming accustomed to them. Although you may still experience some nausea, most women are over that by the end of the fourth month. During this middle trimester, depending on how tall you are, you may begin to 'show', or look pregnant. Some women are so excited to share their news that they even enhance this effect by going early into maternity clothing, or, conversely, continuing to wear snug clothing after it becomes frankly tight so that the 'belly bump' becomes more obvious. Your preference in this matter is your business, and only shows that you are happy and excited to have a baby on board. Now that you are feeling better, and before baby becomes a heavy burden, you are likely to feel more alive than you ever have before, and may literally exhibit that glow that romantic novels talk about. Enjoy it!

Meanwhile, baby is tripling in weight, from about 5 ounces at the end of the fourth month to about a pound and a half by the end of the sixth. Your baby is almost fully developed, although she is not yet ready to make her debut into the outside world. Her skin is smoothing out as she begins to put on the baby fat that makes babies so much fun to cuddle. She still needs more time to complete that process, as well as to finish developing her lungs and other organs for optimal survival. She has hair, fingernails, even eyelashes! If you see an ultrasound picture of her face, you will have an idea of how she will look after birth.

Not so many years in the past, if she were born at the end of the sixth month, your baby would have had no chance for survival. Modern medicine has changed that, saving many babies that are even this premature. Still, a birth at this point is not something to wish for, as many complications make this a very rough road for a new little one. So let's move on to the next trimester with baby firmly and safely ensconced in Hotel Mom.

Third trimester—weeks 30 to 41

As baby puts on more weight, mom begins to feel more fatigued; a natural response to carrying the extra weight. Your fitness level will have even more effect at this point than during the earlier months of your pregnancy. Due to increased pressure on your organs, you may develop the later pregnancy symptoms we mentioned earlier, especially heartburn. Also, your baby is beginning to feel confined, and is punching and kicking as if he could make more room by kicking your ribs out of the way. Oddly enough, this will only amuse you or cause a surge of joy most of the time. Be prepared for the kick to the bladder that has embarrassing consequences, or the one to the ribs that takes your breath away. This vigorous kicking, though sometimes uncomfortable, is a blessing, because you know your baby is alive and well, and anxious to meet the world.

By now, your breasts have fully prepared to nourish your baby, so you may experience leakage of a thick, slightly yellowish substance. If you haven't already done so and intend to nurse your baby, now is the time to invest in a couple of nursing bras and some absorbent pads. You can find both at specialty stores that also carry nightgowns and post-pregnancy tops especially designed to make nursing easy and discreet; nursing pillows to support baby on your lap at feeding time; and other convenience items. Believe it or not, your breasts may grow as much as another cup size or two when your milk fully comes in, but bras that fit now will also fit again later as you begin to wean your baby. It will not hurt to investigate nursing systems that include breast pumps and bottles designed to safely store breast milk, especially if you intend to return to work while still nursing, or suspect that there may be trouble nursing for some reason.

In fact, you will no doubt begin to experience what are termed nesting impulses at this time. Your old friends, hormones, are responsible for preparing you not only physically but mentally and emotionally to be a mom. If you haven't previously set up your baby's own space, whether that is a nursery or a corner of your room, you will have an overwhelming urge to do so now. Women report washing, folding and putting away baby clothes over and over again, arranging and rearranging in an effort to make everything perfect for baby's arrival home. This is harmless, as long as you take care not to inhale paint fumes while decorating the nursery.

If you are fortunate, your friends or family will be planning a baby shower party, where you will receive gifts of baby necessities. If you haven't already done so, you might want to consider registering at local stores for items you particularly want so that your friends will know what to purchase. Doing so before your 36th week will be less taxing on you than waiting until you have to lean backward to keep from falling over on your face from baby's growing weight. Enjoy these parties and preparation time, and be confident that the people who are celebrating with you do so in order to share in your excitement and joy. Everybody loves babies!

While all this preparation is going on, baby is continuing to put on fat stores while putting the finishing touches on her organs, with her lungs being the last to fully develop. Although she can now survive with medical intervention at any point, she is not considered full term until about your 38th week. At any time thereafter, you should welcome a chubby, healthy baby into your anxiously-waiting arms.

Fetal movement

Right along with the joy of knowing you have a baby developing inside you comes the anxiety or frank worry when something changes unexpectedly. It is normal, maybe even inevitable, especially with a first pregnancy when you are experiencing all these changes for the first time. We would venture a guess that every expectant mom and every new mom has had a few anxious moments when she feels that baby is too still

It is unusual for a first-time expectant mom to feel fetal movement before about the 20th week, because up until then the baby is too small to make much of an impact within all that amniotic fluid. Even though you don't feel it, baby is moving quite a bit, and if you were to receive an ultrasound at around the twelfth week, you would see just how much! Between 12 and 16 weeks, movement increases, and women who have been pregnant before or who are particularly attuned to their own bodies might begin to feel sporadic movement by the end of that time. You should not worry that you do not feel movement all the time, because baby still isn't all that active until about 20 weeks.

Around the twentieth week, your baby will begin to increase movement in response to external stimuli, from light to heat and cold. Your own diet and level of activity will play a part, as well. Rhythmic movement, like you would make while taking a walk, might soothe your baby to sleep, just as it will after her birth. But try sitting down or lying down for a nap, and she wakes up, ready to play! That is also the time when you will have more attention to focus on her movements, so they will feel even more pronounced. It is a good idea to begin to get an idea of her sleep cycle and active periods, as these may well carry over after birth. After 20 weeks, you should take some quiet time each day to check your baby's movements, and if you do not feel any for 24 hours, contact your doctor. To stimulate a quiet baby to move, try drinking something cold, like ice water or some cold orange juice. The change in temperature should elicit a response.

From about 29 weeks to about 32, baby's movements will become smaller but stronger. There isn't as much room to move around, but as baby grows stronger, so do his kicks and punches. If you watch your belly, you might see the outline of a little foot cross it as you feel the movement from the inside. This is a never-ending source of entertainment, especially for Dad. Remember, though, that baby is spending a lot of time sleeping, so it won't be constant movement, but should come instead in clusters when he is awake. It is often said that after 32 weeks, movement becomes scarcer, attributed to the tight fit. Pay attention to your own instincts, however. If you become alarmed or overly concerned, call your doctor for a consultation. At the very least, he will be able to allay your fears.

At any time now, your baby will begin to turn head-down and get into birth position, although medical professionals will tell you they have seen babies turn within the last few days, also. Typically, by 36 weeks, baby will be in position and start to descend or 'drop'. When this happens, you will know you are close to delivery! This position may make those kicks more uncomfortable--baby might be able to land one in your ribs or kidneys that will double you over, but it should be more from surprise than painful. Very soon, now, you will be trying to corral those little wriggling legs to change a diaper, and believe it or not, you will miss those inside movements—but not too much, as baby will be in your arms instead.

Labor and delivery

Before your due date—birthing classes

Your doctor will probably provide you with information concerning childbirth classes that will prepare you mentally and physically for labor. Do plan to attend these classes, preferably with a partner who will be your coach during delivery. Your coach can be your spouse, a sister, mother or friend, and it is best to attend the classes with your chosen coach, and a backup coach is not a bad idea. You might be eager to do this as soon as you become pregnant, but talk to your doctor and to friends who have had babies and have attended at different times during their pregnancies. If you are someone who will take the exercises to heart and practice them faithfully throughout your pregnancy, go as early as you would like; but most women will want to attend these classes in the third trimester.

The benefits of taking a birthing class go beyond just knowing how to handle the discomfort of labor. Depending on the type of class you take, you will learn about how your baby is developing, warning signs that something is wrong, how to tell when you are in labor, what to expect during labor and delivery, how to make labor and delivery more comfortable with breathing and relaxation techniques, the role of your coach, how to write a birth plan and more. You may find that your husband feels more included and involved in the pregnancy after taking a birthing class. It is a good place to ask questions and receive support not only from the teacher but from other expectant parents who are taking the classes with you. You may even find friendships there that last beyond the class, and that will provide future playmates near the same age for your little one. Even if the techniques you learn in the class go by the wayside when it actually comes to your own labor, what you have learned will help stem anxiety and allow you to go into labor and delivery with more confidence born of knowledge about the process.

The two most common types of birthing classes in the US are Lamaze and Bradley method. Both of these methods focus on managing pain and stress through breathing and distraction techniques. While the Lamaze philosophy makes no judgments or recommendations about medical intervention for pain, the classes do provide you with knowledge of the options available and their potential risks, so that you can make an informed decision when the time comes. The Bradley method, on the other hand, focuses on avoiding pain medications if at all possible, and emphasizes husband-coached coping techniques. Bradley classes also prepare expectant parents for complications such as emergency C-section. Because the goal of this method is to avoid pain medication, it is the class of choice of parents who opt for home delivery or other non-traditional birthing experience.

Other classes provide alternatives for relaxation and pain management, including yoga and self-hypnosis as a relaxation technique. Choosing the class that is right for you might depend on your husband's willingness to participate, length and duration of the classes, when they are held and how they fit your schedule. You can find classes that last anywhere from five to eight weeks and meet once a week for a couple of hours to two-day weekend classes. To find out your options, ask your obstetrician or midwife, community health organization, hospital or search the internet for local classes. You can also look for classes offered by private childbirth educators, national childbirth education organizations (such as Lamaze International) or even on DVD.

Before your due date—birth plan

A birth plan is nothing more than a written directive concerning your wishes for your childbirth experience. You must understand that it is not a binding agreement between you and your medical provider, as there are too many variables that may have to be accommodated. But writing one does give you the opportunity to really think about what is important to you in this experience. It also helps you communicate your wishes in case your chosen medical professional is not available at the time you go into labor.

A birth plan covers three areas: how you would like to be cared for during normal labor and delivery, how you would like your baby to be cared for immediately after delivery, and what you want to happen in case of unexpected events. In preparing to write this plan, you will need to communicate with your caregiver about your options and choices, as well as the hospital or other venue where you expect to give birth. You may discover that some of your preferences are incompatible, and that is where you will discover what is most important to you. Do you absolutely love your obstetrician, but she will not attend a home birth? Which is more important to you?

Here are some ideas to help you get started:

What do you want to happen during a normal labor and delivery?

How you want to handle pain relief? Will you keep your options open regarding an epidural, or do you want one as soon as it is possible to have it? Think about the environment of the labor and delivery areas, who you want there, what you will be doing while in the early stages of labor, and what birthing methods or positions you would like to use.

How do you want your baby to be treated immediately after birth?

Do you want your partner to cut the baby's umbilical cord? Do you want your baby placed on your stomach immediately after birth if possible? Do you want to try to nurse the baby immediately? Do you intend to breast or bottle feed? Would you like the baby to sleep in the room with you or in the nursery?

Hospitals have a wide variety of policies for newborn care — you will want to know what they are if you plan on delivering at a hospital, how they match what you are hoping for, and whether there is any flexibility.

What do you want to happen in the case of unexpected events?

Of course you do not want to think of something going wrong, but the fact is that C-section delivery is on the rise, so it is better to consider what you want to happen in case your doctor recommends it during labor or in case of other complications. Ask your doctor or midwife what to expect if your labor does not progress after a reasonable period of time, if the fetal monitors indicate your baby is in distress, or about anything else that concerns you. Here more than anywhere else in your birth plan, circumstances might take away your choices, but at least you will have made your wishes known so that your doctor can take them into account to the extent possible.

A discussion of these subjects earlier in the pregnancy rather than later is essential, especially if there are circumstances of your pregnancy that are unusual. You may find that certain wishes are inadvisable because of your age, health or other complications. As your pregnancy progresses, your plan may have to be revised for the same reasons. The process can even help you make a judgment about your caregiver. If he waves off your wishes or concerns and refuses to discuss them with you, you may even want to switch to a provider who is more forthcoming and more understanding of your wish to be completely involved in the planning of your childbirth experience.

Pre-labor symptoms

If you have availed yourself of the childbirth classes that are recommended, you will recognize this discussion as a review of what to expect in the last couple of weeks or days before delivery. If you haven't yet taken a childbirth class and there is still time, we recommend you do so.

First, what is NOT pre-labor! Sometime during the final trimester (although it can rarely happen during the second) your body will begin to experience irregular uterine contractions lasting typically from 30 to 60 seconds and occasionally up to two minutes. These contractions can vary in intensity from merely interesting but not painful to somewhat painful. Most commonly, they are simply uncomfortable. Called Braxton Hicks contractions after the doctor who described and differentiated them from real labor in the mid-1870s, they are unpredictable, irregular in intensity, infrequent, non-rhythmic and do not increase in frequency or intensity. All these characteristics differentiate them from real labor, which has the opposite of each characteristic.

It is believed that these contractions play a part in toning the muscles of the uterus in preparation for the main event, and if they occur during the time that the cervix is dilating and thinning for delivery, they may help that process. A few triggers are mother or baby activity, when someone touches mom's abdomen, after sex, and dehydration. To alleviate the discomfort, you can try changing positions, taking a warm bath for 30 minutes or less (not after the mucous plug has dislodged, discussed below) or drinking a couple of glasses of water, warm milk or herbal tea. If they become very uncomfortable or painful and the steps we have suggested do not alleviate the pain, you should discuss it with your physician.

The first real sign of pre-labor is the event commonly called 'dropping' or 'lightening', wherein your baby prepares for her arrival by descending toward the birth canal. Hopefully, prior to the descent, she will turn head-down in the proper position for birth, but do not be too concerned about this, as doctors report babies turning as late as a few hours before birth. Sometimes the drop can be subtle enough that you do not notice, but your spouse or other close friends and family members might comment that you are holding yourself differently or walking differently because the weight of the baby has repositioned from high and tucked in, to low and forward. You might also notice low back pain or strain due to the baby's weight pulling your spine forward, or possibly groin or hip joint pain because of the weight of the baby pressing on nerve bundles in those areas. This event can occur anywhere from six weeks before delivery to much closer, and baby will continue to descend slowly until the day of delivery when she enters the birth canal and makes her way into the outside world.

A few words about birth position are warranted here. Occasionally, baby will drop into the lower pelvis in a less than optimal position, anything from feet down to rear-end down, to sideways. This is known in general as breech position, and these days most breech babies are delivered by scheduled C-section. The risks of a breech delivery include injury to baby or mom as well as oxygen deprivation to baby if the umbilical cord descends first and therefore gets pinched closed while baby is still relying on it to deliver oxygen. It used to be that massage and other techniques were employed to turn the baby prior to delivery, but those techniques really did not work well, and doctors are now leery of lawsuits for risky deliveries. The risks of C-section are much lower than in previous decades and are considered to be less than the risk of delivering a breech baby vaginally. Now that fetal monitoring by ultrasound is so common, it is less likely that you will have to have an unscheduled C-section for this reason, although other occurrences can create the need for one.

The cervix can begin dilating and thinning (called effacement) as early as a couple of weeks before delivery, or can start the process in the last few days or hours before delivery. As the cervix begins to dilate the mucous plug that has developed to seal the cervix and protect the pregnancy from the introduction of contaminants and bacteria from the outside world will dislodge. This event may be accompanied by 'pink' or 'bloody' show, which is typically caused by small blood capillaries on the surface of the cervix rupturing with dilation. This is not a cause for concern unless there is frank bleeding, in which case you should contact your physician immediately. Both the dislodgement of the mucous plug and the dilation and effacement of the cervix come right before labor itself, but the timing varies from individual to individual.

If you have not already prepared your plans for transport to the delivery facility, packed a bag with everything you will want with you during labor and to bring your baby home with you and let your birth coach know your plans, it is time to do so at this point. You might want to plan your route to the delivery room, and check on alternate routes in case of traffic delays. You will typically have plenty of time to do this, especially with a first baby, once your contractions have started, so don't panic if you have not prepared ahead of time. On the other hand, you will be quite busy timing your contractions and managing your discomfort once labor starts, so it is a good idea not to leave these preparations to the last minute.

First-stage labor

Your labor may start with a few contractions that feel different from the Braxton Hicks contractions you have been experiencing. Or it may get started with the rupture of the placenta, typically known as your water breaking. Even in the latter case, there could still be some hours or even a few days before labor contractions start, although you should notify your doctor when the placenta ruptures whether or not your contractions have started. Most doctors do not want you to have what is known as a dry delivery, so if your contractions don't start within a few hours of the placenta rupturing your doctor may wish to give you a medication to encourage labor.

Assuming contractions start first, your doctor will probably tell you to wait until they are five minutes apart, regular and increasing in intensity before making your way to the delivery room. 'Normal' labor begins with the contractions occurring further apart than that and then settling down at about that interval to a steady pattern of decreasing time between contractions and increasing intensity. However, as you may have guessed, 'normal' is a theory, not what most women experience. Do not feel you are bothering your provider if you are uncertain of what you are experiencing and want some guidance about arriving at the delivery facility and turning your care over to the experts, especially with a first baby.

If at any time before your contractions settle into a pattern and are coming five minutes apart or less (more if you have a long drive to the delivery facility) you experience vaginal bleeding that is more than a trace or if your placenta ruptures and the fluid discharged is a greenish or brownish color, you must get medical help immediately. Unless a hospital is very close and you have someone with you, you would do best to call an ambulance and then your physician. Other than those emergency signals, or labor advancing so quickly that the five-minute intervals become two minutes or less before you can get to your delivery facility, you can expect some hours of labor at home before you are ready to deliver. Of course if you have decided to deliver at home and have no emergencies to change your mind, your midwife is unlikely to arrive before that magic five-minute interval timing. Even when planning a home delivery, you should discuss with your physician or midwife what will happen if you do have an emergency that requires a more sterile environment or a greater level of care than you can receive at home.

As your contractions start, it is not uncommon for them to be spaced as many as 20 to 30 minutes apart. You may not even realize this is the real thing until you have had a few of them, but you will soon understand what is happening, especially if your water breaks during this time. While your contractions are spaced this far apart, you can continue your normal activities and may just have to pause for breath during the contraction itself. There are many anecdotes about what women have done during first-stage labor, from staying at work to mowing their lawns! You might find that what you choose to do becomes a favorite story when your baby is old enough to ask about her birth.

As labor progresses, the time between contractions becomes shorter and shorter and the length of the contraction becomes longer, until, by the end of this stage, the contractions are only two to three minutes apart and might last as long as a minute to a minute and a half. This means there are only seconds between contractions for your body to rest, and that your mind will be fully occupied with what is happening. It is not uncommon to experience other physical symptoms, like shaking or even vomiting. Don't worry, these symptoms are normal, if unpleasant, and do not signal that there is something wrong. Concentrate on managing your discomfort as much as possible. If your doctor agrees, there may be some pain relief medications or other type of pain relief that can help.

The length of time between your first contraction and the end of stage one can vary greatly. First-time moms tend to have the longest labors, and be aware that it can be up to eighteen hours or even more. These days, many doctors will intervene medically if it is taking that long, so be sure to discuss with your doctor under what circumstances you would want that to happen, and how long you would want to labor before it happens assuming your baby is not unduly stressed. It is particularly difficult to make a sensible decision if you are having to listen to your doctor's explanation in 10-second intervals between contractions. Most modern delivery facilities, whether it be a hospital, birthing center, or something else, have fetal monitors that will alert your health-care professionals if your baby begins to be distressed. This is an emergency situation that must be addressed despite any plans you may have, and you may rest assured that if it happens, you will be thinking of the baby first.

Stage-one labor officially ends when you are fully dilated and cleared to push.

Stage-two labor

Although you may have felt the urge to push before being fully dilated, your medical professionals will do their best to prevent you from doing so. This is also one of the points of childbirth classes—how to resist that urge until it will be effective. Pushing your baby down against a cervix that isn't fully dilated will only be frustrating for you and potentially cause injury, so avoid pushing until you are told you may.

On the other hand, some women do not feel the urge, usually due to an epidural or other regional anesthetic. In this case, there is debate about the most beneficial option. Some hospitals and doctors will urge the mother to perform a technique called purple pushing, that involves her holding her breath and forcefully pushing during a contraction, without necessarily feeling the need to do so, to a count of ten. Others, particularly those who advocate for more natural childbirth techniques argue that this does not really help, and that your body is naturally going to push the baby down the birth canal as contractions take place. As long as the baby isn't in distress and you are willing to take this slower route, it is in fact a less-tiring method than the other. It is your choice, in consultation with your doctor, so be sure to discuss it beforehand.

It is at this stage also that some doctors will perform an episiotomy to avoid a perineal tear, or a tear in the tissues around the vaginal opening as they stretch to accommodate baby's emerging head. Once again, there is some debate about the advisability of an episiotomy, which takes about three months on average to heal. One could argue that it is better than a tear, which would also require stitches afterward and might take even longer to heal. On the other hand, there are a few other options that might be more desirable.

Perineal massage, either in the month before labor to help mom learn to relax her pelvic floor and allow the stretch to occur naturally, or during labor to assist the stretching, is one option. Another type of perineal massage provides support to the tissues by pressing against the stretch to prevent tearing. If any of these is the choice you prefer, be sure that your care provider is familiar with the technique and agrees with the concept. Hot compresses help and many women appreciate them for the comfort they provide as well as the assistance in stretching of the area. However, some experts express concern that the area will 'overstretch' the tissues.

Second-stage labor is much shorter than the typical time frame of first-stage, but can last up to four hours, particularly if you have asked your doctor to give you no time limits on pushing. However, many doctors will prefer to move things along as much as possible, to avoid stress on your baby and avoid exhausting you! After all, unless you are in a hospital where you have the option of turning baby over to professional care while you get some rest, you are going to have some major responsibilities very soon after she is born. Assuming everything is proceeding normally, after your baby's head 'crowns' or passes through the vaginal aperture to the point where the forehead and back of the head are visible, the rest of the baby slips out in almost anticlimactic fashion, at least as far as your body is concerned.

The doctor or midwife will quickly clear baby's airway and get him breathing, although the traditional slap to the buttocks is not currently accepted practice. That moment when you first hear your little one's squall of protest at the cold and light of the outside world is one of the most magical times in your life, releasing a flood of hormones that most people recognize as love. Various rituals, such as daddy cutting the umbilical cord, baby being placed in mom's arms or on your chest have grown up around this moment, and with good fortune you may indulge in any of them that your doctor agrees to. However, be patient if medical staff need to work with your baby for a while before you get to hold him. They are doing things that need to be done for his health and welfare, like putting drops in his eyes to prevent infection and taking a small blood sample for a PKU (phenylketonuria—a rare condition in which baby is born without the ability to break down the amino acid phenylalanine) test. These procedures are generally required by law and are done because these diseases are life-threatening but preventable.

Technically speaking, you are no longer in labor, but there is another stage to be endured.

Third-Stage Labor

Although baby has arrived, you must still expel the little apartment she has resided in for the past nine months...the placenta. It was still attached to your baby by the umbilical cord at birth, but the umbilical cord has been cut and baby is now a separate little human being. The placenta in most cases is still inside your uterus, and must be expelled for you to begin recovering from your pregnancy. Normally there will be a few more contractions, taking at most an hour, which will do so. Occasionally there will be complications, but they are usually easy for medical staff to deal with, so this is the real anticlimax. Once the placenta has been delivered, you are done with labor and are now officially a mom!

Postpartum

The word postpartum refers to the period of time shortly after giving birth and is most often used as an adjective to describe any of several complications that can occur during this period. We are using it in the general sense of the time starting with just after delivery and continuing until you are at home and feeling comfortable about caring for your baby.

Immediately after delivery if you are in hospital you and baby may be whisked away separately to be cleaned up, given clean clothes and bedding and made comfortable. Baby will also be weighed and measured, and may have other care done as required (the PKU test may be done at this time, for example). A pediatrician, who may not be the one you have chosen to care for your baby's health needs long term but rather a hospital employee, will check him over to assure his general health and will report to you any problems or concerns that may prevent you from having your baby with you for the time being. Most often your baby will pass his newborn tests with flying colors.

If you have elected to have your baby cared for in your room, he will most likely be brought to you in a hospital bassinette, which often looks like a clear plastic tub placed atop a rolling cart.

Beneath on a shelf will be diapers, baby wipes and other items to care for your baby. Whether you stay for only a few hours while hospital staff ascertains you are both stable or for a few days in the case of a c-section, you may want someone with you to help care for your infant until you go home. Even if everything about labor and delivery are perfect and so is your baby's condition, you will undoubtedly be tired from what is after all a physical ordeal. Take this time to rest and allow others to help if that luxury is available to you. In hospitals where this is not an option, your baby will be cared for by pediatric nurses in the common nursery. These days most hospitals allow mom and baby to bond from as soon after birth as possible, but even when the hospital rules require baby to be in the nursery for the most part, you can ring for your baby to be brought to you to be nursed or bottle-fed as soon as he is deemed stable and ready.

Baby blues, postpartum depression and postpartum psychosis

Most moms can't wait to get home with their babies, where they can cuddle and care for their babies to their hearts' content. Some moms, though, find themselves unaccountably sad after baby is born, one of the common complications we mentioned at the beginning of the chapter. A mild case of teariness, feeling overwhelmed and trouble sleeping combined with being very happy about the baby is known as 'baby blues.' This condition is natural and understandable given the work your body has done and the long anticipatory period during your pregnancy. It usually lasts only a couple of weeks. Good sleep, exercise and nutrition help greatly, so do your best to get these, even though you may be overwhelmed with the care your baby needs. Sleep when baby sleeps, ask for help and be sure to get baby out for a walk in nice weather as soon as her doctor approves.

 If you feel sad, worthless and hopeless for no reason for a long time after your baby is born, you may be suffering from postpartum depression. This condition interferes with your enjoyment of your new baby, and can even be dangerous so by all means contact your physician for assistance in coping with it. Treatment consists of counseling and sometimes medication, although counseling alone is sometimes enough. Some herbal supplements can help, but if you are breastfeeding make sure you have medical opinion before taking anything.

Occasionally postpartum depression can be severe, slipping into postpartum psychosis, which definitely needs intervention. Others may notice that you are acting strangely or seeing things that aren't there. If you find yourself having thoughts of harming yourself or your baby, tell someone right away and get help before tragedy strikes.

Postpartum perineal care

If you have had a vaginal delivery, you may have had a tear of the perineum or an episiotomy. This is a wound, which must be kept clean while it heals. You will likely be discharged from hospital with some equipment that includes a peri-bottle, which is a small bottle with an open tip in the lid used to apply a stream of water to the affected tissues after urination or a bowel movement. This helps clean the area, as well as being a comfort if urination is painful in the first few days, which is common. Pressing a clean pad to the wound during bowel movements will help avoid straining of the tissues and possible re-tearing. You can also soothe the wound with witch hazel pads, found at most pharmacies, placed between the wound and the sanitary pad you will use during postpartum bleeding.

Be prepared for postpartum bleeding, which is the sloughing of the endometrium (the lining of the uterus that has cushioned and worked with the placenta to nourish your baby during pregnancy). It is very similar to a period, but may be both heavier and darker as well as continuing longer than a regular monthly period. During this time you may also experience some cramping, which is due to contractions that are helping your uterus both slough the lining it no longer needs and return to near its pre-pregnancy size. There is no special care needed, but most doctors do not recommend the use of tampons, instead recommending sanitary pads. Although there is no cause for alarm if you occasionally pass small blood clots, contact your health care provider if you soak a sanitary pad within an hour while lying down, pass clots larger than a golf ball, if the discharge has a foul odor or if you develop a fever of 100.4F.

Some new moms experience hemorrhoids or pain upon moving their bowels, especially after a prolonged labor. Soaking in a warm bath, witch hazel pads or topical hemorrhoid medications can relieve these symptoms. A high-fiber diet to keep stools soft will also help—choose fruits and vegetables, whole grains and be sure to get plenty of water. Exercise can also help. As a last resort, ask your physician about a stool softening medication or laxative. On rare occasions, the opposite problem, fecal incontinence, can occur. Frequent Kegel exercises can help, but if you have persistent trouble in controlling your bowel movements, contact your physician.

Postpartum care after C-section

Except for perineal care, everything in the sections above are applicable also to women who have had a C-section birth. In addition, you will have an incision that requires the same care any other incision would, that is making sure no infection develops by keeping it clean and dry. You will be given instructions before leaving the hospital in the case of a C-section, but also keep a few common-sense items in mind. For the first couple of weeks at a minimum, take it easy. Abdominal surgery is no joke, and can cause significant discomfort and fatigue. Try to keep everything you will need close at hand if you are caring for baby by yourself after returning home. Avoid lifting anything heavier than your baby, and in fact if someone else can do that lifting for a while, even better. Rest, rest and more rest is best for the first couple of weeks. Support your abdomen by holding it with your hands or a pillow if you need to cough, sneeze or make other sudden movements, even laughing. Take pain medication as needed—most of it is safe even for breastfeeding moms. Drink plenty of water for all the reasons previously named, especially to avoid constipation as the strain of a hard bowel movement will hurt even more if your abdomen has an incision. Watch for signs of infection, and call your health care provider if the incision is red, swollen or leaking discharge, if you have a fever higher than 100.4F, or if there is increased pain around the incision.

When we discuss breastfeeding in the next section, we will mention that abdominal contractions often accompany it for the first few days or weeks. This may be particularly uncomfortable after a C-section, but try to persist with breastfeeding anyway. You may also have to experiment with positioning baby for breastfeeding. Pillows designed to support baby during breastfeeding should be of great assistance for the C-section mom.

Sex after pregnancy

Most doctors recommend waiting four to six weeks after birth to allow your cervix to close, perineum or c-section incision to heal and vaginal discharge to end. More often than not, mom will not be ready before that due to sheer exhaustion and postpartum discomfort in any case. However, you should know that you may set your own timeframe, and if you feel ready before that it is fine to resume intimacy as long as you make accommodation for any discomfort. Understand that there can be changes, including stretched vaginal muscles reducing pleasurable friction or dryness that is attributable to hormonal shifts (especially if breastfeeding). Kegel exercises can help with the former, and lubricants with the latter. When you do resume sexual intercourse, remember that unless you want to become pregnant right away you must have a reliable method of birth control, even if you are breastfeeding. While it is common for breastfeeding to suppress ovulation, many a mom of 'Irish twins' can attest to the fact that it is also common for it not to.

If you just don't feel like having sex, remember to maintain intimacy in other ways, by cuddling, spending time alone with your partner while someone else cares for baby, and in the countless other ways that characterized your courting period before marriage. You may have to make time between feedings and diaper changes, and dad might be feeling just a little left out as mom and baby bond with breastfeeding, but try to maintain focus on the two of you during these times, rather than worrying about laundry, diapers and baby's other needs. It may feel to one or both of you that sex and intimacy are things of the past, but as long as you acknowledge the changes and make an effort to stay close, they will return eventually.

Breastfeeding

The benefits of breastfeeding have been well established, so only a brief mention of why you would want to do so is required. Mother's milk is specially designed to provide just exactly the nutrition that baby needs for up to the first year of life. In addition, it imparts important immunities until baby is old enough to withstand the risk of disease or be vaccinated. It is convenient, requiring neither special equipment nor refrigeration, sterilization or any of the other inconveniences of formula. It is always available (within certain limits). It even helps mom recuperate from pregnancy by stimulating contractions that help return the uterus to its normal size and expel the endometrium. It is Nature's way. A full discussion of breastfeeding would require a book of its own, and in fact you would be well-advised to acquire one if you intend to breastfeed.

There are also valid reasons NOT to breastfeed, and you might find that one of them prevents you from nursing despite your best intentions. If you did intend to breastfeed, this could be an emotional roadblock, but we will explore some of the reasons to help reduce the emotional pain.

Inverted nipples

This is one of the most common difficulties of breastfeeding, frustrating both mom and baby as baby fails to latch on. The nipple is intended to be erect for breastfeeding, providing the proper shape for baby to take into her tiny mouth. When it turns inward instead, baby can't create the suction to start the flow of milk. Devices called breast or nipple shields are sometimes used to simulate the erect nipple, but lactation specialists generally prefer to show mom how to stimulate the erection manually if possible. Occasionally the inversion is so severe that nothing helps, in which case breastfeeding may have to be abandoned. To help baby receive as much benefit as possible, try a breast pump to extract mother's own milk for bottle-feeding.

Postpartum depression or psychosis

If severe postpartum depression occurs, the pressure to breastfeed can actually be counterproductive and worsen the symptoms. In this case, it is probably best to abandon breastfeeding and provide emotional support to the mom. Formula babies can and do grow up to be healthy, so no guilt should be placed on the mom for not breastfeeding, especially in this circumstance.

Contagious or infectious disease/requirement for unsafe medication

Obviously in the case of contagious or infectious disease, baby should not be exposed through close contact with mom. In the case of chronic illness, medications that mom requires to be as healthy as possible can often be unsafe for baby, who would in this case be better off with formula.

Insufficient milk supply or quality

Occasionally, for many reasons, including poor nutrition on mom's part, the milk supply is insufficient to satisfy baby or promote growth. In this case doctors often recommend supplementing baby with formula to provide the missing nutrition or volume.

Supplementing with formula is a slippery slope, as baby's demand is what increases mom's milk supply, so it often results in the supply shrinking even more. However, if supplementation is required because baby is not gaining weight, it is obviously better to go to formula than to starve the baby.

Summary

Like pregnancy, labor and delivery themselves, the postpartum period soon fades into insignificance as you become more and more comfortable with caring for your baby, watching her develop and integrating her into your family. While there are a few inconveniences and discomforts, you will soon be feeling normal both physically and emotionally, putting it all behind you. At this point, you will no doubt be ready to recover your pre-pregnancy body and concerned to help your baby develop physically, mentally and emotionally.

Remember to also have a look at my **Pregnancy Nutrition** book that contains more than 60 healthy and nutritious recipes for breakfast, lunch, dinner and desserts. You can find the book on my Amazon author page here http://amazon.com/author/john-mcarthur

Bibliography

Murkoff H, Eisenberg A and Hathaway S 1984. What to Expect when You're Expecting.

Simon and Schuster: Kingsway, London. The Baby Blues

Pregnancy and Childbirth: Overcome your Fears and Convert it into Joy.

Pregnancy Guide: Guide to Preparing for Parenthood

Encyclopedia of Natural Medicine Revised 2nd Edition: Michael Murray N.D. and Joseph Pizzorno N.D.

Alternative Medicine: The Definitive Guide; Second Edition: Larry Trivieri, JR Editor, Introduced by Burton Goldberg.

Alternative Cures: Bill Gottlieb

More Books by John McArthur

Hypothyroidism

Hypothyroidism: The Hypothyroidism Solution. Hypothyroidism Natural Treatment and Hypothyroidism Diet for Under Active Or Slow Thyroid, Causing Weight Loss Problems, Fatigue, Cardiovascular Disease. John McArthur (Author), Cheri Merz (Editor)

Fibromyalgia And Chronic Fatigue

Fibromyalgia And Chronic Fatigue: A Step-By-Step Guide For Fibromyalgia Treatment And Chronic Fatigue Syndrome Treatment. Includes Fibromyalgia Diet And Chronic Fatigue Diet And Lifestyle Guidelines. John McArthur (Author), Cheri Merz (Editor)

Yeast Infection

Candida Albicans: Yeast Infection Treatment. Treat Yeast Infections With This Home Remedy. The Yeast Infection Cure. John McArthur (Author)

Heart Disease

Hypertension - High Blood Pressure: How To Lower Blood Pressure Permanently In 8 Weeks Or Less, The Hypertension Treatment, Diet and Solution. John McArthur (Author)

Cholesterol Myth: Lower Cholesterol Won't Stop Heart Disease. Healthy Cholesterol Will. Cholesterol Recipe Book & Cholesterol Diet. Lower Cholesterol Naturally Keep Cholesterol Healthy. John McArthur (Author), Cheri Merz (Editor)

Heart Disease Prevention and Reversal: How To Prevent, Cure and Reverse Heart Disease Naturally For A Healthy Heart. John McArthur (Author)

Diabetes

Diabetes Diet: Diabetes Management Options. Includes a Diabetes Diet Plan with Diabetic Meals and Natural Diabetes Food, Herbs and Supplements for Total Diabetes Control. Delicious Recipes. John McArthur (Author), Corinne Watson (Editor)

Diabetes Cooking: 93 Diabetes Recipes for Breakfast, Lunch, Dinner, Snacks and Smoothies. A Guide to Diabetes Foods to Help You Prepare Healthy Delicious ... Diabetic Meals and Natural Diabetes Food) John McArthur (Author), Corinne Watson (Editor)

Stress and Anxiety

From Stressful to Successful in 4 Easy Steps: Stress at Work? Stress in Relationship? Be Stress Free. End Stress and Anxiety. Excellent Stress Management, Stress Control and Stress Relief Techniques. John McArthur (Author)

Anxiety and Panic Attacks: Anxiety Management. Anxiety Relief. The Natural And Drug Free Relief For Anxiety Attacks, Panic Attacks And Panic Disorder. John McArthur (Author), Cheri Merz (Editor)

Back and Neck Pain

The 15 Minute Back Pain and Neck Pain Management Program: Back Pain and Neck Pain Treatment and Relief 15 Minutes a Day No Surgery No Drugs. Effective, Quick and Lasting Back and Neck Pain Relief. John McArthur (Author)

Arthritis

Arthritis: Arthritis Relief for Osteoarthritis, Rheumatoid Arthritis, Gout, Psoriatic Arthritis, and Juvenile Arthritis. Follow The Arthritis Diet, Cure and Treatment Free Yourself From The Pain. John McArthur (Author)

Depression

How to Break the Grip of Depression: Read How Robert Declared War On Depression ... And Beat It! John McArthur (Author)

Pregnancy

Pregnancy Nutrition: Pregnancy Food. Pregnancy Recipes. Healthy Pregnancy Diet. Pregnancy Health. Pregnancy Eating and Recipes. Nutritional Tips and 63 Delicious Recipes for Moms-to-Be. Corinne Watson (Author), John McArthur (Author)

Pregnancy and Childbirth: Expecting a Baby. Pregnancy Guide. Pregnancy What to Expect. Pregnancy Health. Pregnancy Eating and Recipes. Cheri Merz (Author), John McArthur (Author)

Allergies

Allergy Free: Fast Effective Drug-free Relief for Allergies. Allergy Diet. Allergy Treatments. Allergy Remedies. Natural Allergy Relief. John McArthur (Author), Cheri Merz (Editor)